CARCINOGEN

Edited by **Margarita Pesheva, Martin Dimitrov**
and **Teodora Stefkova Stoycheva**

Carcinogen

Edited by Margarita Pesheva, Martin Dimitrov and Teodora Stefkova Stoycheva

Published by InTech

Janeza Trdine 9, 51000 Rijeka, Croatia

Publishing Process Manager Romina Skomersic

Technical Editor Teodora Smiljanic

Cover Designer InTech Design Team

Additional hard copies can be obtained from orders@intechopen.com

Carcinogen, Edited by Margarita Pesheva, Martin Dimitrov and Teodora Stefkova Stoycheva
p. cm.
ISBN 978-953-51-0658-6

For EU product safety concerns:
IN TECH d.o.o., Prolaz Marije Krucifikse Kozulić 3, 51000 Rijeka, Croatia,
info@intechopen.com or visit our website at intechopen.com.

Meet the editors

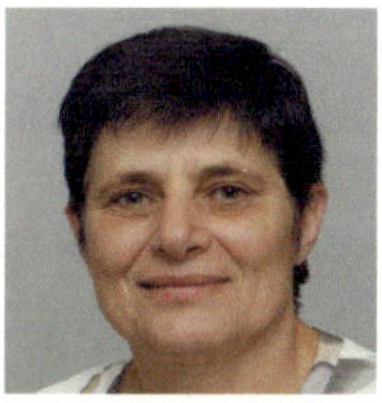

Assoc. Professor Margarita Pesheva is the leader of the Laboratory of microbial genetics at the Department of Genetics, Sofia University. She received her M.Sc. from Sofia University, Bulgaria and Ph.D. from the University of St. Peterburg, Russia. Dr. Pesheva gives lectures and practical exercises in Genetics, specifically Bacterial Genetics and Genetics and selection of microorganisms. During the last years, the scientific interests of Dr Pesheva have focused on construction of yeast strain *Saccharomyces cerevisiae* with gene modified Ty1 retrotransposon. Dr Pesheva is the co-author of "Tool for Quantitative Determination of Antioxidant Activity of Different Natural Products in Alive Cells".

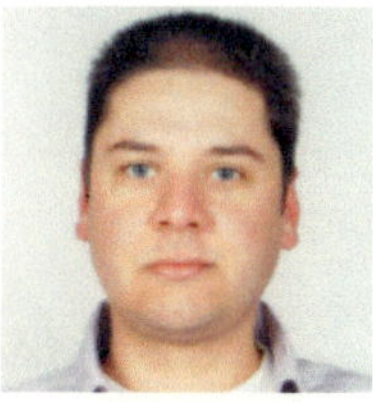

Dr M. Dimitrov defended his Ph.D. thesis at the Department of Genetics, Sofia University. His research interests are focused on revealing the molecular mechanisms of carcinogenic action of different laboratory carcinogens, environmental pollutants and food improvers, and understanding the role of carcinogen-induced ROS levels as activators of Ty1 transposition in yeast *Saccharomyces cerevisiae.*

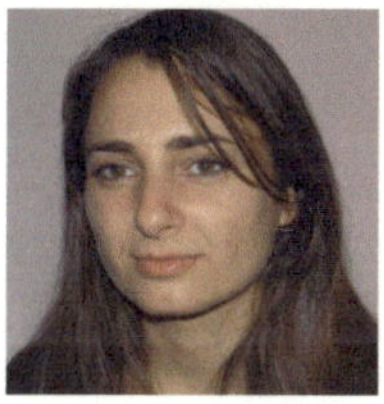

Dr Teodora Stefkova Stoycheva defended her Ph.D. thesis in Thermophysics and Hydrodynamics. Her research interests are focused on revealing the molecular mechanisms of carcinogenic action of different laboratory carcinogens, environmental pollutants and food improvers, and understanding the role of carcinogen-induced ROS levels as activators of Ty1 transposition in yeast *Saccharomyces cerevisiae.*

Contents

Preface

During the last decades, cancer diseases have increased all over the world. The low quality of food and strong pollution of environment are the main prerequisites for carcinogenesis. The main problem for scientists is to find strategy for prevention of cancer diseases. Therefore, the information about models for studying carcinogenesis and mutagens which appear during cooking, environmental pollutants, and tests for specific detection of carcinogens is particularly important.

The book "Carcinogen" contains a collection of reviews and original papers which illustrate:

Models of Carcinogenesis - a review focused on the role of stem cells as target to carcinogenesis

Tests for Detection of Carcinogens - one of the reviews describes different methods for analyzing nucleic acid adducts, while the other describes the Ty1 retrotransposition short-term test, which can be used to study carcinogenicity of chemicals, including such applied in agriculture, nutrition and pharmacy. The test is highly sensitive, selective to carcinogenic substances, and can be used to control environmental pollution.

Food and Carcinogens - one of the reviews gives general information about mycotoxins. Some of them have biological effect on human health, the others, however, are carcinogenic according to their mechanism of action. The quality of food depends on the heat treatment during cooking process, which may cause the formation of mutagenic and carcinogenic compounds. Food industry has to monitor and control food technology to ultimately reduce food born carcinogens.

Environmental Carcinogenesis - four reviews are closely focused on environmental pollution with carcinogens and their effect on human health - the risk of leukemia arising from formaldehyde exposure, the effects of bisphenol A (BPA) exposure to cancer risk, the consumption of high amount of water containing humic acid, and genome instability caused by ionizing radiation. The book "Carcinogen" is intended for biologists, researchers, students in medical sciences and professionals interested in associated areas.

Dr. Margarita Peshev
Sofia University, Faculty of Biology, Department of Genetics,
Bulgaria

Dr. Martin Dimitrov
Sofia University, Faculty of Biology,
Bulgaria

Dr. Teodora Stefkova Stoycheva
Institute of Cryobiology and Food Technology,
Department of Cryobiology and Lyophilization,
Bulgaria

Section 1

Model of Carcinogenesis

The New Model of Carcinogenesis: The Cancer Stem Cell Hypothesis

Brenda Loaiza, Emilio Rojas and Mahara Valverde
Universidad Nacional Autónoma de México, Instituto de Investigaciones Biomédicas
México

1. Introduction

Cancer has long been seen as a disease that arises from mutations and epigenetic alterations that impair the capacity of any cell within the organism to deregulation its proliferation, avoid apoptosis and metastasis, giving rise to malignant transformation. Progressively, these early cancer cells lead to different generations of daughter cells that accumulate additional mutations, acting in concert to drive the full neoplastic phenotype. Adult stem cells are found in numerous tissues of the body and play an important role in tissue development, replacement and repair. In addition, these cells show long-term replicative potential, together with the capacities of self-renewal and multi-lineage differentiation. These stem cell properties are tightly regulated in normal development, therefore their alteration may be a critical issue for tumorigenesis. The Cancer Stem Cell (CSC) theory arises from the poor probability of short-lived differentiated progenitors or terminally differentiated cells to accumulate mutations that become cancer. On the other side, the normal tissue stem cells or early progenitors that already possess the most important characteristics of cancer are an easy target for the accumulation of genetic aberrations which lead to cancer formation. The new defining model for carcinogenesis, the "cancer stem cell theory" was put forward since 1997, when John Dick and coworkers started a series of pioneering investigations to understand whether the functional hierarchy observed in normal hematopoiesis was conserved in blood tumors (Bonnet & Dick, 1997). According to this model cancer is a stem cell disease that places malignant stem cells at the centre of its tumorigenic activity. Cancer stem cells give rise to undifferentiated cells and terminally differentiated cells, as happens in normal tissue renewal, but the major difference between cancer growth and normal tissue renewal is that whereas normal transit amplifying cells usually differentiate and die, at various levels of differentiation, the cancer transit-amplifying cells fail to differentiate normally and instead accumulate (ie, they undergo maturation arrest), resulting in cancer growth.

Cancer stem cells may be caused by transforming mutations and/or epigenetic events to gain the self-renewal activity and lose some features of differentiation occurring in multi-potential stem cells, tissue-specific stem cells, progenitor cells, mature cells and cancer cells. This theory has been functionally supported by the observation that among all cancer cells within a particular tumor, only a minute cell fraction has the exclusive potential to regenerate the entire tumor cell population. Many groups have extrapolated the cancer stem cell theory from the haematopoietic system to solid cancers, where using in vitro culture techniques and in vivo transplant models have established evidence of cancer stem cells in colon, pancreas, prostate, brain and breast cancers. Some tumor stem cells, like breast, have upregulated genes which include Notch. Notch signaling has been highlighted as a pathway involved in the development of the breast and is frequently deregulated in invasive breast cancer, as well as other oncogenic pathways like Wnt, Hh and NF-κB. Also studies on haematopoietic cancers show that these important signaling pathways for normal haematopoiesis, are oncogenic, thereby potentially involved in cancer stem cell regulation.

On the other side, the degree of differentiation of a carcinoma depends on the proportion of undifferentiated tumor stem cells. The cancer-derived differentiated cells are not normal, moreover they don't have the potential to develop cancer, so it could be attempt to direct normal differentiation of malignant stem cells and serve as an alternative to cytotoxic therapy. Differentiation therapies are currently underway. To be maximally effective, therapy of cancer must be directed against both the resting stem cells and the proliferating cells of the cancer. Conventional radiation treatment and chemotherapy only kill the actively proliferating cells of the cancer. Successful therapies could be reached if specific stem cell signals are inhibited using gene therapy, while at the same time attacking proliferating cells by conventional radiation treatment or chemotherapy. However, the chemoresistant phenotype of CSCs makes it difficult to increase their sensitivity to anticancer drugs and to decrease the rate of cancer recurrence in patients that is the one of major causes of death all over the world.

This review will focus on the role of stem cell as a target to carcinogenesis, the major oncogenic pathways and finally provides an update of the major chemoresistance related mechanisms of cancer stem cells.

2. The raise of the stem cells

At the dawn of the 20th century, we had recognized that chemicals cause cancer, but we had not yet identified individual cancer-causing molecules, nor did we know their cellular targets. What we lacked was knowledge of the mechanisms by which chemicals cause cancer and the molecular changes that characterize tumor progression. We now are early in a century in which cancer is being investigated at the molecular level, and we have developed technologies that afford unprecedented power to delineate and manipulate altered pathways in cancer cells (Loeb & Harris, 2008). However we still been confronted with the same old kind of questions and realities, Can we harness new insights and technologies to prevent or obliterate human cancers or delay their progression? Can we give more specific molecular-based therapeutic options to a cancer patient? Can we identify the origin of the carcinogenesis process?, defining these questions is a critical step to a complete understanding of carcinogenesis.

In the last 15 years a great advance has been performed trying to understand the mechanisms underlying the origin of the carcinogenesis process. With the concept of stem cells the cancer scenario suffers an extraordinary expansion. Nowadays with the discovery that almost all tissues in the body are able to renovate owing to the presence of Stem Cells (SCs), most of medical research about regeneration therapy involve the study of these cells. Indeed when looking for stem cells in Pubmed there are more than 150,000 papers. Since

1961 with Till and McCulloch initial work, lot of researchers have dealt of isolating and identify stem cells in all tissues (Till & McCulloch, 1961).

Stem Cells are defined principally by its genuine capacity of self-renewal, as a matter of fact in assays for identification of stemness is necessary to demonstrate this property. Some of most popular assays to evaluate functionally are, in the case of hematopoietic stem cells (HSC), the long term repopulating of the entire hematopoietic system of myeloablated animals *in vivo*. These studies have been done by transplanting murine HSC into irradiated, SCID (severe combined immunodeficient) and NOD/SCID (non-obese diabetic/severe combined immunodeficiency) mice (Jordan & Lemishka, 1990; Kamel-Reid & Dick J, 1988). Immunophenotypic analysis and functionally *in vitro* are, also, carry out to identify stem cells, for example, HSC are defined by their capacity to initiate and sustain long-term hematopoiesis in liquid cultures in presence of an adherent cell layer formed by stromal elements (Sutherland et al., 1990).

As responsible of the tissue renovation, SCs have an extraordinary expansion potential and an important capacity of differentiation, giving rise to a heterogeneous hierarchical progeny of cells (Mayani, 2003). To produce differentiated cells and at the same time preserve the stem cell pool, stem cells undergo asymmetric or symmetric cell divisions. Asymmetry division refers to two different daughter cells; a stem cell and a progenitor cell capable of differentiating, meanwhile, symmetric cell divisions contribute to regulate cell pool size giving rise to two identical stem cells, or two progenitor cells. In certain cases such as in hematopoiesis, it is likely that both mechanisms operate to preserve the SCs pool and give rise to all the different lineages and maturation stages (Mayani et al., 1993).

SCs types generated during development are the fertilized egg, or zygote, which is by definition the "Totipotent" stem cell capable of produce all the different cells of an organism, including those that do not form part of the embryo, such as placenta cells (Alberts et al., 1994, Wobus, 2010). Totipotent stem cells are up to morula (8-cell) stage, each cell produced is identical to the zygote. Then the embryo becomes blastocyst, in which each cell that forms part of the inner cell mass is capable of producing all cells of the embryo itself, but not extraembryonic structures produced only by trophoblast cells that then become placenta. At blastocyst stage, each cell is a "Pluripotent" Embryonic Stem Cell (ESC) with an unlimited proliferation potential (Williams, 1988). Three types of pluripotent stem cells lines with self-renewal capacity and the potential to differentiate into cell types of all three primary germ layers were derived from embryos and fetal stages of mice: embryonic stem (ES) cells were isolated from blastomeres of the early mouse embryo from the 8-cell up to the blastocyst stage (Evans & Kaufman, 1981, Wobus et al., 1991); embryonic germ (EG) cells were isolated from primordial germ cells, the precursor cells of germ cells from 9.5- to 12.5-day fetal stages (Resnick et al., 1992); and embryonic carcinoma (EC) cells have been established from the stem cell population of teratocarcinomas (Figure 1). These three cell types share typical characteristics, such as expression of alkaline phosphatase, the embryonic antigen SSEA-1 (Solter & Knowles, 1978) and the germline-specific transcription factor Oct-4 (Scholer at al., 1989), a short G1 phase of the cell cycle (Rohwedel et al., 1996) and high telomerase activity (Thomson et al., 1998).

A novel source of stem cells is induced pluripotent stem cells (iPSC) and adult multipotent stem cells. iPSC cells were first derived from murine fibroblasts by ectopic expression of

Oct4, Sox2, Klf4 and c-Myc transcription factors, demonstrating that the specialized somatic cells can be reversed into a pluripotent state in vitro (Takahasi & Yamanaka, 2006). Like embryonic stem (ES) cells, iPSC cells are able to self-renew indefinitely and to differentiate into all types of cells in the body. iPSC hold great promise for regenerative medicine, because iPSC avoid immunological rejection but also get away from ethical issues (Chen & Liu, 2009). Since the first report on the derivation of iPSC in 2006, many laboratories all over the world started research on iPSC cells and have made significant progress.

In the other hand, Till and McCulloch (1961) were the first to detect spleen-colony forming units in mouse bone marrow and to realize that these were a kind of stem cell, since that time, stem cell for a number of other adult tissues have been identified. The fundamental role of adult stem cells in a living organism involves maintaining the somatic cell population in tissues in response to cellular injuring or stress, and thus such stem cells are important in maintaining tissue homeostasis in the organism. Adult stem cells are multipotent differentiating into a few cell types, usually limited to the tissue from which they arise, however, a few reports have suggest that have the potential to differentiate to cells other than their tissue of origin (Charbod, 2010; D´lppolito et al., 2004; Jiang et al., 2002) (Figure 1).

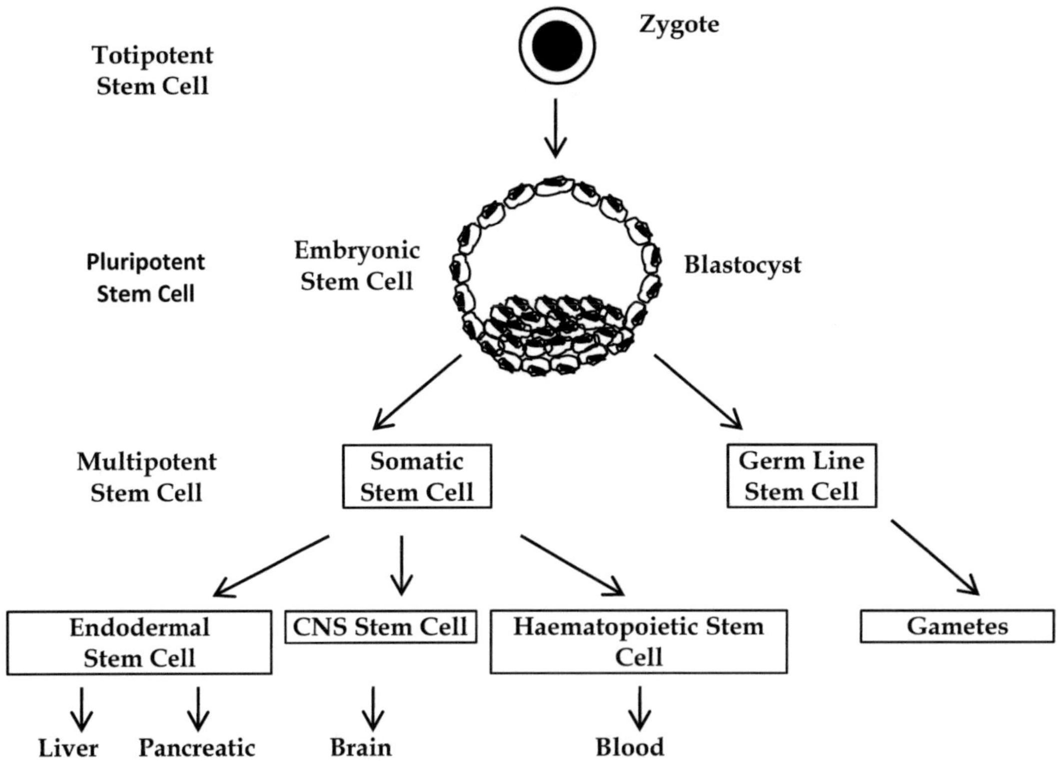

Embryogenesis starts with the fertilized oocyte, zygote (totipotent stem cell), which develops into embryonic stem cell (pluripotent stem cell). Somatic and germ line cells represent the multipotent stem cells. CNS: Central Nervous System.

Fig. 1. General Types of Stem Cells.

Stem cells develop within specific microenvironments called "niches" consisting of different cell types and their products, these external elements provide signals that control stem cell behavior by modulating expression and activity of the nuclear transcription factors, gene expression, molecular regulators of cell cycle, epigenetic regulation, etc., (Oh & Kwon, 2010). To avoid aberrant growth or tissue loss, the balance between stem cell proliferation and differentiation must be perfect. In natural conditions, stem cells are found in quiescence and their frequency is very low (Orford & Scadden, 2008). For example in bone marrow, where are located the vast majority of HSC, there are 1 HSC per 1–2 x 10^4 bone marrow cells (i.e., 0.01–0.005% of total bone marrow cells) (Szilvassy & Hoffman, 1995; Thomas et al., 1999), and as we have mentioned previously, the location of HSC within the bone marrow is not random. Most HSC are located within the endosteal region, whereas lineage-committed progenitors and mature cells are distributed away from this region, predominantly in the central marrow region, close to the central marrow vessels (Nilsson et al., 2001).

In the elegant manuscript of the hallmarks of cancer, Hanahan and Weinberg (2011) described a set of events necessary to reach a transformation condition, it was worth-noting for a lot of researchers that some of these events are present in stem cells, because these cells can undergo extensively cell division and has the potential to give rise to both stem cells and cell differentiate into specialized cells, opening the possibility of the participation of stem cells in cancer process. The still unresolved question is how stem cells, which stay in very well maintained niches, interacts with environmental factors that provide them the damage that will became an irreversible deregulated self-renewal? How oncogenes and/or tumor suppressors genes can be compromised in cancer stem cell process?

2.1 Stem cells as target of mutations and transformation

Target cells of transforming mutations is unknown, even in cancer; however there is considerable evidence that certain types of leukemia arise from mutations that accumulate HSC. This proposal is sustained in the fact that cells capable of initiating human Acute Myeloid Leukemia (AML) have a $CD34^+CD38^-$ phenotype in most AML subtypes and thus have similar phenotype to normal HSC. Conversely, $CD34^+CD38^+$ leukemia cells cannot transfer disease, despite the fact that they exhibit leukemic blast phenotype. This suggests that normal HSC rather than committed progenitors are target for leukemic transformation (Reya el at., 2001).

In a work of Miyamoto an colleges (2000), done on HSC from patients in remission, AML1-ETO transcripts which result of the most frequent chromosomal translocation 8;21 were found in a fraction of normal HSC in the marrow. These prospectively isolated HSC and their progeny were not leukemic, indicating that translocation occurred originally in normal HSC and that additional mutation in a subset of these HSC or their progeny subsequently lead to leukemia. Other evidences where clonotypic leukemia-associated chromosomal rearrangements have also been found in $CD34^+CD38^-$ lymphoid (George et al., 2001) and chronic myeloid leukemias (Mauro & Druker, 2001).

Although SCs are often target of genetic events that trigger malignant transformation, in other cases restricted progenitors or even differentiated cells may become transformed. Mouse model in which myeloid leukemia arises from restricted progenitors was created by targeting the expression of transgenes specifically to restricted myeloid progenitors using the hMRP-8 promoter, this model of leukemia resemble human leukemias in many respects. The enforced expression of anti-apoptotic gene bcl-2 in the myeloid linage leads to a disease that is similar to human chronic myelomonocytic leukemia, including monocytosis, splenomegaly and neutropenia, as the mice age, but rarely these mice develop acute malignancies. To test whether additional mutations are required to synergize with bcl-2 to promote AML, hMRP8-bcl-2 transgenic mice were bred with lpr/lpr Fas-deficient mice. Remarkably, the loss of these two distinct apoptosis pathways led to the development of AML in 15% of the mice (Traver et al., 1998). These mice have an expansion of myeloblast in all haematopoietic tissues, with substantially lowered number of granulocytes in the marrow and blood. As previously described, in the case of spontaneously arising human leukemias it is likely that stem cells accumulate the mutations that are necessary for neoplastic proliferation; however these mutations are expressed in restricted progenitors. That is, mutations that accumulate in stem cells may lead to neoplastic proliferation of primitive progenitors downstream of stem cells. Perhaps the reason why only 15% of mice progress to AML expressing Bcl-2 and lacking Fas is that the progenitors in these mice also must acquire an additional mutation that cause deregulated self-renewal. If a single additional mutation causes transforming events is probably a gain-of-function mutation, such as one that promotes constitutive self-renewal. Due that stabilized β-catenin promote self-renewal of HSCs and other progenitors, Reya and colleges (2001) propose that gain-of-function mutations in β-catenin may, transform deathless pre-malignant cells to cancer cells by promoting proliferation.

2.2 Evidences about the existence of Cancer Stem Cells (CSC)

The first's evidences about the existence of Cancer Stem Cells were documented for leukemia and multiple myeloma reporting that only small subset of cancer cells is capable of extensive proliferation. When leukemic cells were transplanted in vivo, only 1-4% of cells could form spleen colonies (Bruce & Van der Gaag, 1963; Wodinsky et al., 1967). Even when mouse myeloma cells were obtained from ascites, separated from normal hematopoietic cells and put in clonal in vitro colony forming assay, only 1 in 10,000 to 1 in 100 cancer cells were able to form colonies (Park et al., 1971). The clonogenic leukemic cells were described as leukemic stem cells because the differences in clonogenicity among the leukemia cells mirrored the differences among normal haematopoietic cells. Bonnet and Dick (1997) show that human Acute Myeloid Leukemia (AML) stem cells could be identified prospectively and purified as $CD34^{+}CD38^{-}$ cells form patient samples. Despite the fact that these cells represent only 0.2% of variable proportion of AML cells, they were the only cells with the capacity of transferring AML from human patients to NOD/SCID (non-obese diabetic/severe combined immunodeficiency) mice in the vast majority of cases. For solid tumors, also has been shown that the cells are phenotypically heterogeneous and that only a small proportion of cells are clonogenic in vivo and in culture; for example, in lung cancer, only 1 in 1000 to 1 in 5000; ovarian cancer and neuroblastoma cells were found to form colonies in soft agar. Only in terms of leukemic stem cells, these findings led to the hypothesis that only a few cancer cells are actually tumorigenic and that these tumorigenic cells could be considered as cancer stem cells (CSC).

In most human breast cancer, only a very small fraction of the tumor clone defined as $CD44^{+}$,CD24neg/low and representing 11-35% of total cancer cells, is able to sustain tumor grow when xenografted in NOD/SCID mice (Al-Hajj et al., 2003). The CSC working model has also been proved in brain tumors, Galli et al., (2004) succeeded to isolate and propagated neurospheres from human glioblastoma, which are highly enriched in long-term cell renewing multi-linage-differentiating and tumor-initiating cells. Another example for demonstrating the existence of CSC was found in rapidly renewing intestinal cells (small intestine and colon). This epithelium is full with normal stem cells localized at the bottom of the crypts and expressing the Wnt target gene Lgr5. Stem cells that were disrupted of the APC (Adenomatous Polyposis Coli) gene were leading to constitutive activation of the Wnt pathway, a well known initiation step in intestinal cancer. The result was the formation of microscopic adenomas, a first step in malignant transformation of the intestine. Interestingly, when the APC gene was deleted in more differentiated and short-lived progenitors, microadenoma could be observed that however lacked growth potential and did hardly result in microscopic adenoma formation (Lapham et al., 2009).

2.3 Theory of cancer stem cell

In cancer biology has long recognized that tumor is complex collections of aberrant cells, each of which ultimately derives from a single antecessor, the cell of origin that describes their clonal source. The process by which the cell of origin develops into an ever-expanding, heterogeneous tumor that retains many features of its parent tissue remains mysterious. In this classical carcinogenesis model, a somatic differentiated cell had to be reprogrammed or "dedifferentiated" to regain immortalization properties of cancer. The limited life span and proliferation capacity of the differentiated cell should be induced to an irreversible change that enables the cell to get the ability to have unlimited proliferation (Trosko, 2009); then after, this initiated cell have to survive long enough to acquire the hallmarks of cancer. Recently the cancer stem cell theory has re-emerged as a compelling model to explain both the clonality and some of the heterogeneity of tumors. It postulate that each tumor contains a subset of cells, cancer stem cells, that are unique responsible for tumor growth, heterogeneity and metastasis. These cells specialized; possess important features, self-renewal and differentiation potential, that together pointing out them from the remainder of the tumor cells (Rothenberg and Clarke, 2009).

The cancer stem cell theory proposes that tumors have a cellular hierarchy that is a caricature of their normal tissue counterpart because they reflect the pluripotency of the originally transformed cell.

Two observations lead to this theory, first most tumors arise from a single cell, but not all the cells in a tumor are identical this is also known as tumor heterogeneity (Park et al., 1971). A widely held belief in cancer biology is that all cellular heterogeneity found in tumors may be attributed to genomic instability and the selection for cells that can adapt to the tumor microenvironment. However recent evidence strongly supports that CSC also plays a major role in tumor heterogeneity (Lobo et al., 2007).

The second observation was build came from studies that demonstrated that a large number of cancer cells were required to growth a tumor (Bruce & Van der Gaag, 1963; Hamburger & Salmon, 1977). Two formal possibilities could explain this observation: either all cancer cells had a low probability of proliferating extensively or most cancer cells were unable to proliferate extensively and only a small, definable subset of cells was consistently clonogenic.

In both cases, some of the cancer cell heterogeneity would arise a result of environmental differences within the tumor and continuing mutagenesis. The essential difference between these possibilities is the prediction, according to the second possibility that whatever the environment or mutational status of the cells, only a small phenotipically distinct subset of cancer cells has the ability to proliferate extensively or form a new tumor.

The cancer stem theory postulate that only some tumor cells, cancer stem cells, are tumorigenic. When they divide, these malignant cells self-renew, and also give rise to the non-self-renewing cells that go on to elaborate the heterogeneous cells within a cancer. In this sense, CSC´s both drive tumor growth, and also initiate the execution of a developmental program. Cancer stem cells thus utilize pre-existing developmental hierarchies, and give rise to some of the cellular heterogeneity seen in such tumors.

After proposal of cancer stem theory, the term "cancer stem cell" is an operative definition that does not necessarily connote a developmental relationship to normal stem cells; instead, it merely states that a subset of cells within a tumor can self-renew and elaborate tumor heterogeneity. Recently, the definition depends on the assay of self-renewal and tumorigenicity. Also, the cancer stem cell theory does not imply what percentage of cells within a tumor are cancer stem cells. Some very aggressive tumors may have a high percentage of CSC´s (Kelly et al., 2007, Kennedy et al., 2007), and chemotherapeutic treatments may increase the frequency of CSC´s in a tumor (Dylla et al., 2008); however neither of these observations affects the operative definition. Is important to mention that stochastic model and the cancer stem are not mutually exclusive. Since they are malignant cells, CSC´s likely exhibit genomic instability, and have a mutator phenotype (Hannahan & Weinberg, 2000). Thus, as they divide and give rise to both tumorigenic and non-tumorigenic progeny subclones of CSC´s may develop.

2.4 Proposal of cancer stem cell model integration into the stochastic model

It is believed that the initiation step is caused by a mutation or any other irreversible event, in which the single normal cell acquire an advantage proliferation capacity and/or to avoid apoptosis. Given the natural characteristics of stem cells, the initiation process could be more easily carry out if the cell has per se the capacity of self-renewal, then to complete the step, only the deregulation of these mechanisms would be needed, a good example of this is the aberrant activation of the Wnt signaling pathway in many cancer types and especially those of the gastrointestinal tract. Indeed, Wnt signaling activity was shown to designate colon CSCs (de Sousa et al., 2011).

On the other side, promoting conditions can be wound healing, surgery, cell death, inflammatory agents, growth factor hormones, and mutagenic or non-mutagenic chemicals that stimulate proliferation, then, the initiated cell must be clonally expanded, process which also can be facilitated by self-renewal and great proliferation properties of stem cells. It is important to highlight that in most of the tumors it has been seen blocked differentiation, so the initiated cell would not terminally differentiate and neither die by apoptosis (Piscaglia et al., 2007). Indeed, if we begin the transformation with a stem cell rather than with a differentiated cell, the block of differentiation process would be easier that reprogramming or "dedifferentiation, consequently, in promotion step the adult stem cells inhibits its ability to complete differentiation under normal conditions and the symmetric division is preferred, meanwhile any other normal stem cell would divide preferentially in the asymmetric way to favor differentiation, and could die by apoptosis or suffer senescence if any damage is not resolved (Reviewed in Trosko, 2009)(Figure 2).

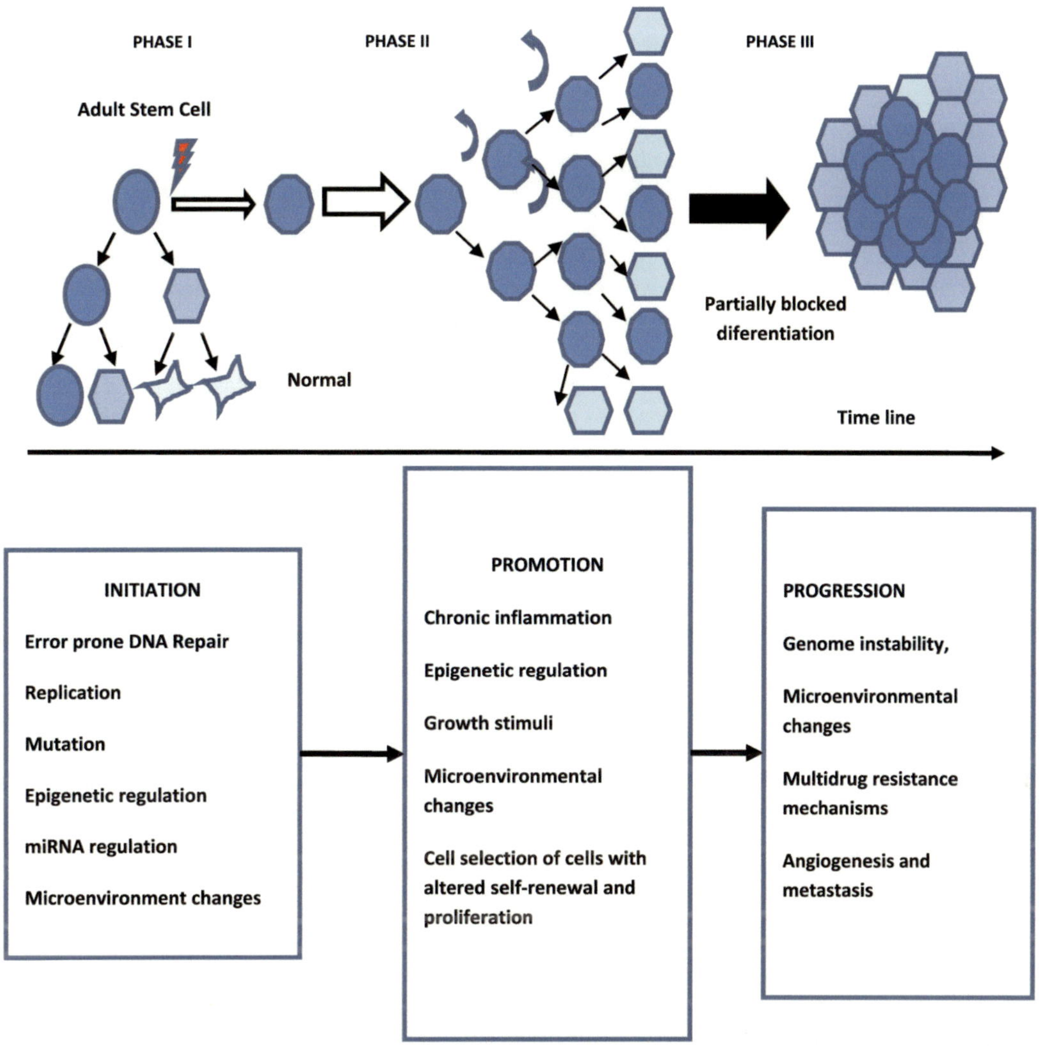

Fig. 2. Integration of the Cancer Stem Cell model into the stochastic model of carcinogenesis.

The stochastic model of carcinogenesis process consists of 3 principal steps. The first one is the initiation process, which had to irreversibly convert a normal somatic differentiated cell to a premalignant state. The second step is the promotion stage, where the single initiated cell is clonally expanded by a mitogenic process, and is unable to die, even if the microenvironmental conditions favorite apoptosis. The last step, the progression, has traditionally seen as the process when the tumor completes its malignant transformation and become metastatic. Cancer stem cells may be caused by transforming mutations and/or epigenetic events, to gain the self-renewal activity and lose some features of differentiation occurring in multi-potential stem cells, or progenitor cells. This model has been functionally supported by the observation that among all cancer cells within a particular tumor, only a minute cell fraction has the exclusive potential to regenerate the entire tumor cell population. Many groups have extrapolated the cancer stem cell model from the hematopoietic system to solid cancers, using in vitro culture techniques and in vivo transplant models; they have established evidence of cancer stem cells in colon, spleen, prostate, brain and breast cancers.

Finally, when the expanded initiated cells accrue sufficient alterations to become growth stimulus independent, and resistant to growth inhibitors and apoptosis, to have unlimited replicative potential and invasive and metastatic phenotypes, then the progression phase has been achieved (Trosko et al., 2004). About stem cells, some of these have *per se* the properties unlimited replicative potential, as wells as the homing capacity, passing inadvertently all over the organism, and also plasticity, to change their phenotype (Figure 2). Given is well known these processes also, enable metastasis, a program involved in various steps of embryonic morphogenesis and wound healing called "epithelial-mesenchymal transition" (EMT), has been recently implicated in metastases. Cells which suffer EMT acquire stem cells phenotype and the abilities to invade, to resist apoptosis, and to disseminate.

2.5 Evidences that not all cancer cells are tumorigenic

Under the CSC´s model, only a subset of cells is capable to self-renew and generate at least part of a tumor´s developmental heterogeneity, other malignant cells within the tumor should be non-tumorigenic. A number of independent observations, both in the clinic and basic research level needs to take in account to be clear that tumor are heterogeneous cell populations.

The most startling experiments in cancer biology are of Southam and Brunschwig in 1966. At that time, physicians had realized that malignant cells could be found circulating in the blood or lymphatic of cancer patients, but only small percentage of these seemed to give rise to metastatic tumors. Southam and Brunschwig sought to test this observation directly by harvesting tumor cells of patients with various disseminated or unresectable cancer, dissociating tumor fragments into single cell suspensions, and then subcutaneously autotransplanting varying number of cells to roughly determine how many tumor cells were needed to generate a new tumor (Southam et al., 1966). In spite of the deep ethical and methodological flaws, this study did suggest that, using their methods, only a subset of cells within a tumor is tumorigenic. Similar findings have being documented in different cancer patients, patients with malignant ascites, breast cancer (Braun et al., 2005, Riethdorf et al., 2008), and liver cancer. In the case of cancer patients with malignant ascites who have implantation of peritoneo as procedure which help alleviate abdominal distention, but also has the unavoidable effect of shunting huge number of tumor cells into systemic circulation, disseminated cancer is a rare event (Campioni et al., 1986, Tarin et al., 1984). A related clinical example is the recognition that viable breast cancer cells have been found in the bone marrow of a large percentage of patients. Although in many patients the presence of these cells correlates with an increased probability of overt metastasis and a worse overall prognosis, the vast majority of these cells either remain dormant for years or are simply not tumorigenic (Braun et al., 2005; Riethdorf et al., 2008). Another supportive example is the observation that percutaneous biopsy of breast and liver tumors frequently leads to the disruption of the tumor and the deposition of thousands of malignant cells along the biopsy track, yet even with large bore needles, the rate of tumor seeding of the biopsy track is relatively low (Ryd et al., 1993; Eriksson etal., 1984; Smith, 1984; Diaz et al., 1999). Several possibilities could explain this discrepancy, including the idea that only a fraction of the tumor cells are tumorigenic.

Along these lines, in many different animal models of cancer (both with hematologic malignancies and solid tumors) a large number of tumor cells must be transplanted into a recipient animal in order to generate a tumor. Similarly, only a minority of tumors cells is able to proliferate in vitro and generate colonies (Hamburger & Salmon, 1977a; Hill and Milas, 1989; Cho et al., 2008).

2.6 Return of some tumorigenic cells to nonmalignant cells

The Cancer Stem Cells theory implies that tumor heterogeneity is, at least in part, due to the execution of a developmental program in the progeny of cancer stem cells. As defined, cancer stem cells should be immature, multipotent, and able to give raises both tumorigenic and non-tumorigenic cells. This has been shown in the case of mouse teratocarcinoma, a malignant germ cell tumor that can give rise to differentiated cell types of all three germ layers. When this tumor develops, it will metastasize and kill the host within a matter of weeks. Single cells, when injected subcutaneously into recipient mice, cause tumor to form. However, when single genetically-marked teratocarcinoma cells are isolated and injected into a normal mouse blastocyst, the progeny of the teratocarcinoma cells contribute functioning terminally-differentiated post-mitotic cells to multiple different tissues without inducing more tumors (Mintz & Illmensee, 1975). Importantly, among cancer, teratocarcinomas are not unique in their ability to execute a program of differentiation. Experiments with a transplantable squamous cell cancer in rats showed that tumor growth is driven mainly by immature, proliferating cells that subsequently develop into differentiated cells that, when transplanted, lose their tumorigenicity (Pierce & Wallace, 1971). Also, supportive data in humans comes from the genetic analysis of leukemic clone can also be seen in mature, well-differentiated cells of various lineages. This suggests that the cancer is driven by immature hematopoietic cells that retain the capability of generating mature, noncancerous progeny (Fialkow, 1972; Fialkow et al., 1977).

3. Pathways involved in stem cell deregulation

Cell signaling involved in cancer had been extensively studied in the last decades; several pathways had been involved in this process. Many of the molecular mechanisms underlying tumorigenesis in cancer and self renewal in stem cells have been elucidated in the past decade, but with the introduction of the cancer stem cell theory, the carcinogenesis field began to change the form to look at the pathways involved in this process.

A subtle change in the conceptualization of the illness had been developed in the last years, from our first cancer definition as a cell proliferation problem to an acquirement of stem-like phenotype passing through a dead incapacity problem, the form to deal with this process had been change enormously. Cancer cells have the ability to divide indefinitely and spread to different parts of the body during metastasis. At the other hand embryonic stem cells can self renew and, through differentiation to somatic cells, provide the building blocks of the human body (Dressen & Brinvanlou, 2007). Then it is possible to hypothesizer that certain highly conserved genes may contain evolutionary-conserved self-renewal machinery, and this machinery (at least in part), must be present in both normal and cancer stem cells. Day by day, the study of stemnes genes take relevance in the understanding the circuitry of cancer cells.

Among of the pathways that have been involved in the stemnes phenotype, seven of them seem to be constantly present: cascades of signaling involve Signal Transducers and Activators of Transcription (STAT), Fibroblast Growth Factor (FGF), Tumor Growth Factor (TGF), WNT, Phosphatidylinositol 3-kinase PI3K/AKT, Notch and Hedgehog signaling pathways. Furthermore, the stemnes phenotype is the result of a very well orchestrated and unique gene expression pattern characterized by the activation of some genes and the repression of others. Then, elucidation of the stemnes phenotype is based primarily on the identification of the transcription factors involved in regulating gene expression of the stemnes state (Cavaleri & Schöler, 2009). Among them Oct-4, Sox2, Nanog, NF-kB and recently miRNAs has been involved in this process, for that, in the present section we will discuss their role in carcinogenesis.

3.1 Jak/STAT signaling

Cells can communicate with each other through the secretion of cytokines. After binding their receptors, receptor-associated Janus Kinases (JAKS), as well as interacting Signal Transducers and Activators of Transcription (STATs) through tyrosine phosphorylation form homodimers, shuttle to the nucleus and participate in transcriptional regulation of a variety of genes (Darnell, 2002, 2005). STATs are also activated in response to growth promoting factors such as Epidermal Growth Factor (EGF) or Platelet-Derived Growth Factor (PDGF). Identification of STAT3 as a determinant of ES renewal came from Smith´s and Yokota´s laboratories at the end of 90's, where demonstrated that STAT3 docking sites are essential in mediating transmission of the signal in self-renewing ES cells. Thus, the JAK/STAT pathway plays an important role in mediating cell fates, such as apoptosis, differentiation and proliferation, in response to growth promoting factors and cytokines (Matsuda et al., 1999; Smith, 2001).

Deregulated JAK/STAT signaling can contribute directly and indirectly to tumorigenesis. Mutations, fusions, and/or amplification of JAK/STAT signaling components, such as the HER2/neu- in mammary and stomach carcinomas, or Epidermal Growth Factor-Receptor (EGF-R) in breast, brain and stomach tumors, can confer hypersensitivity to mitogenic signals and promote proliferation (Slamon, et al., 1987; Yarden, & Ullrich, 1988).

Additionally, STAT3 is constitutively activated in several major human carcinomas. Also, STAT3 is persistently active in over 50% of lung and breast tumors and more than 95% of head and neck cancers (Darnell, 2005).

3.2 FGF signaling

Twenty-two FGF family orthologs are conserved among mammalian genomes. FGF dimmers bind to FGF receptors with extracellular immunoglobulin-like domain and cytoplasmic tyrosine kinase domain. FGF signals are transduced through FGF receptors to activated PKC signaling cascade and the $Ca2^{+}$- mediated NFAT signaling cascade. FGF signals are also transduced through FGF receptors and FRS2/FSR3-SHP2-GRB2 docking protein to the SOS-RAS-RAF-MEK-ERK signaling cascade and GAB1/GAB2-PI3K-PKD-AKT signaling cascade. The RAS-ERK had been implicated in cell growth, differentiation and cancer, while PI3K-AKT signaling cascade in the cell survival, cell fate determination and also in cancer.

3.3 TGFβ signaling

The TGFβ superfamily includes nearly 30 proteins in mammals, e.g. TGFβ, activins, nodal GDF, and BMPs. Smad 1/5/8 transduce signals from Bmps, and GDFs ligands, whereas Smad 2/3 transduce signals from TGFβ, activins and nodal. Upon activation by phosphorylation and association with a common Smad4, the receptor-activated Smads translocate to the nucleus to regulate gene expression in concert with other transcription factors (Cavaleri and Schöler, 2009). It has long been appreciated that the TGF-β pathway plays a crucial role during embryonic development. Several lines of evidence suggest that TGF-β signaling is also involved in sustaining the undifferentiated state in hESC. Activin / Nodal branch of TGF-β signaling is necessary to sustain pluripotency. In contrast the BMP branch of TGF-β signaling appears to play the opposite role (Dressen & Brivanlou, 2007). In conclusion, extensive studies established the TGF-β signaling pathway as a major regulator during embryonic development. Mutations or downregulation of TGF-β receptors, inactivation of SMAD4 or p15INK4B can be found in a variety of cancers. BMP2 is dramatically overexpressed in 98% of lung carcinomas (Langenfeld et al., 2003; Langenfeld et al., 2006). TGF-β signaling can also enhance malignancy of epithelial tumors by stimulating metastasis (Hartwell et al., 2006; Yang et al., 2004; Zavadil & Bottinger, 2005).

3.4 WNT signaling

WNT/β- catenin pathway, is associated with many kind of cancers, secreted Wnt ligands bind to frizzled receptors and activate a cascade important in development. WNT signaling increases the expression of HoxB4 and Notch-1 genes. Both of these proteins are implicated in the specification and /or self-renewal of HSCs (Reya et al., 2003). In addition, the Wnt/β-catenin pathway is involved in the maintenance of the normal epithelial cells and in regenerative responses during tissue repair (Reguart et al., 2005).

Wnt signaling has been implicated in blood diseases and colon carcinoma. Activating mutations of β-catenin or inactivating mutations of the adenomatosis polyposis coli (APC) gene, which targets β-catenin for degradation, occur in a large percentage of colon cancers (Kolligs et al., 1999). In CML, β-catenin accumulates in granulocyte-macrophage progenitor cells when CML progresses to blast crisis (Jamieson et al., 2004). β-catenin accumulation has also been associated with breast cancer, melanoma, sarcoma, myeloid leukemia, multiple myeloma, brain tumors and in the other hand, mutations in β-catenin are also observed in endometrial, prostate and hepatocellular carcinomas (Reguart et al, 2005).

3.5 PI3K/AKT signaling

Phosphatidylinositol 3-kinase/AKT (PI3K/AKT) pathway responds to a variety signals, like hormonal receptors, transmembrane tyrosine kinase-linked receptors (RTK) and intracellular factors and has been implicated in the regulation of several processes such as cellular proliferation, cell death and cytoskeletal rearrangements (Hennessy et al., 2005). Activation of PI3K occurs through interaction with various activating proteins such as protein kinase C (PKC), RHO, RAC, mutated RAS, SRC and leads to activation of phosphatidylinositol-3,4,5-biphosphate (PIP3). PI3K/AKT signaling is counteracted by PTEN (and SHIP1, SHIP2), which dephosphorylates PIP3. In the other hand AKT protein kinase interacts with Phophoinositide Kinase 1 (PDK1), and regulates directly or indirectly a number of downstream targets, such as NF-κB, BAD, pro-caspase 9, MDM2, p53 and GSK3.

Deregulated PI3K/AKT signaling has been observed in various cancers. Mutations in the PI3K/AKT pathway inhibitor and tumor suppressor PTEN has been found in glioblastomas, lung carcinomas and melanomas whereas AKT overexpression or overactivation has been found in breast, ovarian, thyroid and a variety of other cancers (Vivanco & Sawyers, 2002).

3.6 Notch signaling pathway

DLL and Jag families are transmembrane-type ligands for the Notch family receptors (Radtke & Raj, 2003). Ligand binding induces the cleavage of the Notch family members by metalloprotease and γ–secretase to release Notch intracellular domain (NICD) for the interaction with CSL or NF-kB transcription factors.

Notch signals are transduced to the canonical CSL-NICD signaling cascade and the non-canonical NICD-NF-kB signaling cascade. HES1, HES5, HEY1 and 2 and HEYL genes, encoding transcriptional repressor with bHLH and orange domains, are target genes of the canonical Notch signaling cascade. The notch signaling activation have been implicated in gastric cancer resulting in the maintenance of stem or progenitor cells through the inhibition of epithelial differentiation (Katoh, 2007).

3.7 Hedgehog signaling pathway

Sonic hedgehog (SSh), Indian hedgehog (IHh) and Desert hedgehog (DHh) are members of the hedgehog (Hh) family of secreted signaling proteins having diverse function during vertebrate development. Hh signaling also functions postembryonically in tissue homeostasis through effects on stem or progenitors cells. Inappropriate activity of the Hh pathway have been linked in pancreatic, skin, brain and gastric cancer and tumor types that arise sporadically or in genetically predisposed individuals. SHh signaling is launched by binding with the transmembrane protein Patched (PTCH) resulting in the loss of the PTCH activity and consequent phosphorylation and post-transcriptional stabilization of smoothened (SMO) protein. Pathway activation via SMO thus can occur either by Hh protein stimulation or through loss of PTCH activity (Ruiz et al., 2002; Tang et al., 2011).

3.8 Regulation factors involved in cancer stem cells gene expression

3.8.1 Oct-4

The Oct3/4 gene, a POU family transcription factor Oct3/4 or Oct4, (also referred to as Pou5f1), was first found in ovulated oocytes, mouse pre-implantation embryos, ectoderm of the gastrula (but not in other germ layers) and primordial germ cells, as well as in embryonic stem cells but not in their differentiated daughters (Rosner et al., 1990).

Nowadays is well known that Oct-4 is also expressed in Adult Stem Cells, where it normally start the terminal differentiation process and when Oct4 gene activity is down-regulated, differentiation of both stem cells and embryonal carcinoma cells occurred (Tai et al., 2004). In addition, it has been shown, that the success or failure of cloning depends on expression of this gene, during reprogramming of the genome of a nucleus transferred to an enucleated oocyte (Boiani et al., 2002). Seemingly in contrast, the Oct4 gene has also been shown to be expressed in some human tumor cells but not in normal somatic tissues.

Also, Oct-4 provides adult stem cells the property to sell-renew and proliferate, so when differentiation process takes place the Oct-4 expression is lost. In Tai´s work (2004), when the human breast epithelial, spleen and liver stem cells were induced to differentiate, Oct4 expression markedly diminished, but when a stem cell is initiated by up-regulation of Oct-4, the cell is able to differentiate and maintain the transcription factor expression and consequently the ability to self-renew occurred. Using antibodies and PCR primers against Oct-4, the group of Trosko, tested human breast, liver, spleen, kidney, mesenchyme and gastric stem cells, as wells as, the cancer cell lines HeLa and MCF-7 and human, dog and rat tumors for evidencing the Oct4 expression. They found that adult human stem cells, immortalized non-tumorigenic cells and all tumor cells tested express Oct-4, but not the differentiated cells (Tai et al., 2005). In addition, with these results, they conclude that adult cells expressing the Oct4 gene could be the target cells for initiation of the carcinogenic process, because they were able to isolate non-tumorigenic, but immortalized clones that exhibited phenotypic markers similar to the original stem cell and, after X-ray irradiation, they could also isolate weakly tumorigenic clones which could be rendered highly tumorigenic after transfection with the c-erb B-2/neu oncogene.

3.8.2 Sox2

Sox2 belongs to the Sry-related HMG box-containing family of proteins that binds to the minor groove of –DNA through the 79 amino-acid HMG domain. Sox2 is a major stemness factor. Indeed, it is a critical transcription regulator of the normal stem cell phenotype of ESCs, with a restricted number of partners, including Oct-4 and Nanog. It controls self-renewal and differentiation processes through coordinated transcriptional programs. As forced Oct4 expression induces pluripotency in Sox2-null cells, a group of researchers concluded that the primary role of Sox2 in induced pluripotent stem cells is controlling Oct4 expression, and they perpetuate their own expression when expressed concurrently. More recent studies indicated that Sox2 exits in the nuclei of ES cells and acts as a transcriptional factor to maintain the unique characters such as clonogenicity, pluripotency, and self-renewal of them (Masui et al., 2007).

A number of links were recently found between Sox2 and cancer; it has been intensively investigated and was found to contribute to the establishment of lung, prostate and spleen cancer (Saigusa et al., 2009, Sanada et al., 2006, Rodriguez-Pinilla et al., 2007).

3.8.3 Nanog

In 2003 Chambers and Mitsui reported the identification of Nanog as a new member of the embryonic stem cell stage. Nanog is a gene expressed in ESCs and is a key factor in maintaining pluripotency. Nanog is thought to function in concert with other factors such as pou5f1 and Sox2 to establish ESC identity. Oct4 and Sox32 control Nanog transcription by binding to this element in both mouse and human ES cells. Overexpression of Nanog in mouse embryonic stem cells causes them to self-renew in the absence of leukemia inhibitory factor. In the absence of Nanog, mouse embryonic stem cells differentiate into visceral/parietal endoderm (Chambers et al., 2003, Mitsui et al., 2003). Loss of Nanog function causes differentiation of mouse embryonic stem cells into other cell types (Lin et al., 2005). Gene knockdown of Nanog promotes differentiation, thereby demonstrating a role for these factors in human embryonic stem cell self-renewal (Zaehres et al., 2005).

Somatic cells respond to DNA damage by activating p53, which causes cell cycle arrest or apoptosis. ES cells, under high levels of DNA damage, lack the p53 dependent G1 arrest and cells undergo apoptosis. However, at low levels of DNA damage, it has been shown that p53 binds to the promoter of Nanog and suppresses its expression in mouse embryonic stem cells. p53 can thus induce differentiation of embryonic stem cells into other cell types which undergo efficient p53-dependent cell-cycle arrest and apoptosis (Lin et al., 2005). Nanog protein has been implicated in several types of cancer such as: bladder, colorectal, gastric, prostate and oral squamous cell carcinoma (Chiou et al., 2008).

3.8.4 NF-kB

Nuclear factor of kB (NF-kB) is a transcription factor involved in the inflammatory and innate immune responses (Lin & Karin, 2007). The activation of NF-kB occurs as it is transported from the cytoplasm to the nucleus upon degradation of the inhibitory subunit. In the nucleus, it binds to specific kB sites on the DNA and mediates the expression of mostly genes involved in the cellular response to stress (Ghosh & Karin, 2002). The REL family proteins of NF-kB form various homo and heterodimers, and their activity is regulated by two main pathways. The canonical NF-kB activation applies to dimers that are composed of RELA, c-REL, and p50, which are held captive in the cytoplasm by specific inhibitors that are known as the inhibitor of kB (IkB) proteins. This pathway is normally triggered in response to microbial and viral infections and exposure to proinflammatory cytokines and physical and chemical stresses. Cellular stresses such as ionizing radiation and chemotherapeutic agents also activate NF-kB (Karin & Ben-Neriah, 2000).

The first link between NF-κB and cancer was when the subunit p50 was identified as a member of the REL family, which is also the family of the famous oncoprotein v-Rel, of the REL retrovirus (REV-T) (Gilmore et al., 2004). Activation of NF-kB is a tightly regulated event, in tumor cells, different types of molecular alterations may result in an impaired regulation of NF-kB activation. In such cases, NF-kB becomes constitutively activated, which leads to deregulated expression of NF-kB controlled genes. According to Hanahan and Weinberg in the hallmarks of cancer NF-kB is able to induce all of cellular alterations that become cancer (Hanahan & Weinberg, 2011).

3.8.5 MiRNA Regulation

Micro RNAs are small, 19–22 nucleotide (nt) long, non-coding RNAs that inhibit gene expression at the posttranscriptional level. The mRNA/miRNA duplex then inhibits translation either through a (mRNA 5') cap-dependent mechanism affecting initiation or through increased degradation of the mRNA. Given the frequency with which miRNA target motifs are conserved within 3'UTRs, it is estimated that 20 to 30% of all human genes are targets of miRNAs, and that for each miRNA hundreds of genes exist that carry conserved sequence motifs within the 3'UTR (Peter, 2009).

miRNAs have been shown to regulate embryonic development (Stefani and Slack, 2008). Upregulation of miRNAs is required for various differentiation processes in fact, little is known with respect to mechanisms by which miRNA function in controlling the developmental potential of ES cells. However, it is still largely unknown how ES cell-specific transcription factors and miRNAs work together (Bar et al., 2008; Calabrese et al., 2007; Mineno et al., 2006).

A strong link between miRNA deregulation and human cancer has been established. A comparison of miRNA expression in normal and tumor tissues demonstrated global changes in miRNA expression in various human malignancies. In addition, mapping of 186 human miRNA genes has revealed that they are frequently located at fragile sites and other cancer associated chromosomal regions. Consequently miRNAs have been demonstrated to act either as oncogenes or tumor suppressors (He et al., 2007; Akao et al., 2006; Zhang et al., 2006; Calin et al., 2004).

4. Cancer stem cells as a target for chemotherapy: The problem of resistance

Despite all the new knowledge and advances in treatment, cancer remains one of the most common causes of death all over the world. Failure in treatment is the principal cause of the mortality, and it could be due to the cancer ability to recur and spread after initial therapies. Relapses may be caused in part to the existence of CSCs. Thus, CSCs are regarded as the root of cancer origin and recurrence. New therapeutic approaches targeting these malignant cells have become the topic of ongoing research. However, the chemoresistant phenotype of CSCs makes difficult to increase their sensitivity to anticancer drugs and to decrease the rate of cancer recurrence in patients.

4.1 Mechanisms of resistance to traditional chemotherapy

The trouble of chemotherapy resistance has been present since 1945, when Gilman and co-workers introduced chemotherapy into clinical practice at the end of the Second World War. They used nitrogen mustard to treat a patient with advanced malignant lymphoma, after an initial regression of the disease, a second course of therapy was given, however a lesser therapeutic effect was observed and after the third treatment, the tumor no longer responded to the agent (Goodman et al., 1946).

The drug resistance can be due to diverse factors: pharmacokinetics, such as inadequate access of the drug to the tumor, inadequate infusion rate and inadequate route of delivery (Garattini, 2007). Another important factor is drug metabolism which can inactivate and efflux the drug. The cytochrome P450 enzymes, a multigene family of constitutive and inducible haemo-containing oxidative enzymes from the liver, play an important role in the metabolism of a diverse range of xenobiotics and are often over expressed in a variety of solid tumors, in which they can contribute to drug resistance. The third factor are the membrane proteins such as solute carriers channels and ATP-binding cassette (ABC) transporters; they can facilitate the drug efflux from the cell, in fact colon and liver cancer have an intrinsic drug resistance, due to the function of these type of transporters, which are already highly expressed in the healthy tissues (Gottesman et al., 2002, 2006).

Mutation or over expression of the drug's target is another mechanism of resistance, for example the case of protein BCR-ABL in CML. The chimaeric BCR-ABL protein is a constitutively active protein tyrosine kinase with an important role in the regulation of cell growth (Melo & Barnes, 2007). Imatinib mesylate (formerly STI571; Gleevec, Novartis, Basel, Switzerland) is a potent and highly specific competitive inhibitor of the BCR-ABL tyrosine kinase. Initially, it had a high rate of cytogenetic and hematologic responses in patients with chronic-phase CML, in whom previous therapy had failed, and actually, its use has revolutionized the management and clinical expectations of CML patients. Unfortunately, not long after its initial use, resistance to Imatinib was demonstrated in CML patients.

Approximately 50% of imatinib-resistant CML patients carry a resistance-associated point mutation in BCR-ABL, which interferes with imatinib binding, and more than 50 different resistance-associated point mutations in BCR-ABL have been seen (Gorre et al., 2001). Also BCR-ABL gene amplification or over expression at the mRNA and protein levels has been detected in clinical samples (Hochhaus et al., 2002). The BCR–ABL fusion oncogene has also been implicated in NF-kB activation, cell survival, and tumorigenesis in human leukemias (Reuther et al., 1998).

As mentioned above, resistance appears not only to traditional chemotherapy but also to targeted therapies such as tamoxifen, which targets the estrogen receptor (ER) in breast cancer (Ali & Coombes, 2002); Imatinib, which targets the constitutively active kinase BCR-ABL important role in the regulation of cell growth (Melo & Barnes, 2007) in CML.

In addition to p53 mutations which inactive the tumor suppressor, p53 pathway can also be inactivated in wild-type p53- carrying tumors, via indirect mechanisms such as MDM2/MDMX amplification. In fact, most wild-type p53 types of cancer harbor alternative genetic alterations such as mutations in APC in colon cancer, BRCA1 and BRCA2 in breast cancer, and B-RAF in melanoma (Soussi & Wiman, 2007).

4.2 The cancer stem cell and drug resistance

The failure to eradicate cancer may be as fundamental as a misidentification of the target. Antitumor treatments designed and selected for broad cytotoxic activity may kill mostly of cancer cells and induce regression of the tumor; however according to the CSC model, cancer stem cells will re-establish tumor growth and cause relapse from therapy. In other words, therapeutic approaches that do not eradicate the CSC compartment are likely to achieve little success (Reya et al., 2001). In fact, the whole drug resistance concept has been revised incorporating the CSC paradigm, and recognizing of stem cells in different tissues, can help to distinguish the degree of damage tolerance and multipotentiality and then translate it into differential drug susceptibilities depending on the tissue of origin (Donnenberg & Donnenberg, 2005).

Current views favor the model that cancer stem cells are innately resistant to chemotherapy through their relative quiescence, their enhanced capacity for DNA repair, decreased entry into apoptosis, and ABC transporters expression. The inherently slow cycling rate of CSCs has been hypothesized to provide them inherent defense against most traditional chemotherapeutic regents, which are antiproliferative and most effectively target the fastest dividing cancer cells (Graham et al., 2002). On the other side, the problem of resistance can be more complex, the expression and activity of ABC transporters is one of the most important markers for stem cells and cancer stem cells, they have high multidrug resistance (MDR) pump activity associated with high expression of the ATP-binding cassette family of proteins such as ABCB1 (P-glycoprotein) and/or ABCG2 (Breast Cancer Resistance Protein-1, BCRP1) (Wu & Alman, 2008).

The well-known, side-population (SP) phenotype is due to the expression of ABCG2 and has been detected in both normal and AML hematopoietic stem cells. In fact, expression of ABCG2 and Hoechst 33342 effluxes are two of the best markers of these cells, interestingly that expression is often turned off during differentiation to progenitor and mature blood cells (Kim et al., 2002). Imatinib is both an ABCG2 substrate, and inhibitor, making it susceptible to efflux by stem cells that express this transporter (Burguer et al., 2004; Houghton et al., 2004).

Imatinib and Gefitinib are, also, both direct and downstream inactivators of ABCG2 and, therefore, serve as candidates to reverse cancer stem cell chemoresistance and potentially target cancer stem cells (An & Ongkeko, 2009). Nevertheless, the level of contribution of ABC efflux chemoresistance and their inhibition remains controversial in clinical trials (Leonard et al., 2003). Unfortunately, there are lots of reasons that make, the ABC transporters, an incomplete and dangerous targeted to finish with the chemotherapy resistance. The expression of ABCG2 by microvessel endothelium of the brain suggests that ABCG2 plays an important role in maintaining the Blood Brain Barrier BBB. Thus, anti-ABCG2 therapy that successfully eliminates ABCG2+ CSCs may lead to adverse neurotoxic effects (Cooray et al., 2002). On the other side, it has been proposed that selective pressure imposed by chemotherapy leads to both mutation and secondary genetic changes, including MDR upregulation in the bulky tumor (Donnenberg, & Donnenberg, 2005).

The redundancy of the individual transporters within the MDR phenotype together with several other resistance-related proteins expressed in solid tumors (eg, glutathione S-transferase, metallothionin, O6-alkylguanine-DNA-alkyltransferase, thymidylate synthase, dihydrofolate reductase, heat shock proteins), may contribute to the failure when inhibiting only the MDR proteins.

4.3 Novel targets against cancer stem cells

In a very recent work for characterization of cancer stem cells in CML, it has been demonstrated that TKI (tyrosine kinase inhibitors) don't function with CSC of CML. First, efflux Hoechst dye, express CD34, lack CD38 and cytokine-non-responsive cells were isolated, and then these cells had been shown to regenerate bcr-abl-positive haemopoiesis in immunocompromised mice upon transplantation. CML stem cells express very high levels of functional wild-type bcr-abl; however, no kinase domain mutations were detected in the stem cell population. FTIs (farnesyl transferase inhibitors) have activity against CML. BMS-214662 was the most effective of these and induced apoptosis of phenotypically and functionally defined CML stem cells in vitro, as a single agent and in combination with IM or Dasatinib. In association with apoptosis, there was activation of caspase 8 and caspase 3, inhibition of the MAPK pathway, IAP-1 (inhibitor of apoptosis protein-1), NF-kB and iNOS (inducible nitric oxide synthase) (Jorgensen & Holyoake, 2011). Fumitremorgin C (FTC) is derived from the fermentation broth of *Aspergillus fumigates* and was the first specific ABCG2 inhibitor. FTC is a potent inhibitor of ABCG2 and has been shown to reverse mitoxantrone-resistance in selected cancer cell lines (NeRabindran et al., 1998). Moreover, neurotoxicity has precluded the clinical use of FTC. Inhibitors of ABCB1 are already in clinical use, some of these compounds also effectively target ABCG2, including Elacridar (GF120918) and Tariquidar (XR9576) (Robey et al., 2004, 2007).

Another field of research in the resistance is directed at the identification of pathways known to be involved in the regulation of growth and self-renewal properties of CSCs, such as the Wnt, Notch and Hedgehog (Hombach-Klonisch et al., 2008).

4.4 Role of NF-kB in chemotherapy resistance

The role of the canonical NF-κB pathway in mammary tumorigenesis was investigated using a transgenic (TG) mouse expressing a dominant-negative inhibitor of kappaB (IkappaB alpha(SR (S32A/S36A))). TG and control mice were subjected to a chemical carcinogenesis protocol. Hyperkeratinized squamous metaplasias, were found in both TG and control mice. p65/RelA- and NF-κB DNA-binding activity were detected in mammary luminal lesions, but rarely in squamous metaplasias. Analysis of NF-κB family proteins and target genes using microarray data from a cohort of human mammary tumors revealed the expression of a canonical NF-κB pathway, but not non-canonical pathway proteins in HER2+ luminal cancers. HER2+ tumors also showed differential regulation of specific NF-κB target genes relative to basal and ER+ luminal cancers. Isolation of mammary cell populations enriched for stem and progenitor cells by fluorescence-activated cell sorting and with the help of an NF-κB-EGFP reporter mouse, demonstrated that luminal progenitors contain activated NF-κB whereas the mammary stem cell-enriched population does not. Together these data suggest that the canonical NF-κB pathway is active in normal luminal progenitor cells before transformation and is required for the formation of mammary luminal-type epithelial neoplasias (Pratt et al., 2009).

As we have reviewed in this study, the NF-κB pathway is a major source of pro-inflammatory cytokines, which may contribute to cancer chemoresistance. Constitutive NF-κB activity has been observed in ovarian cancer stem cells (OCSCs). Leizar and coworkers used Eriocalyxin B (EriB) for the inhibition of NfκB and induction of cell death. OCSCs and mature ovarian cancer cells (mOCCs) were treated with increasing concentrations of EriB, and then, cell viability was measured, caspase activity and cytokine levels were quantified. EriB decreased the percent of viable cells in all cultures tested with GI(50) of 0.5-1 μm after 48 hrs of treatment and induced cell death by inhibition of NF-κB activity, EriB produced decreased cytokine levels and activation of caspases, too. Down-regulation of XIAP and sensitizing of OCSCs to TNFα and FasL-mediated cell death were others effects of EriB (Leizer et al., 2011).

In a very recent work, with the fact that Disulfiram is a specific inhibitor of ALDHs and, therefore, it may also be an inhibitor of Breast Cancer Stem Cells (BCSCs), Wang's group used Disulfiram (DS)/copper and inhibited BCSCs and enhanced cytotoxicity of paclitaxel (PAC) in Breast Cancer (BC) cell lines: MCF7, MDA-MB-231 and T47D. The constitutive NF-kB activity in BC cell lines was inhibited by DS/Cu. Combination index isobologram analysis demonstrated a synergistic effect between DS/Cu and PAC. The increased Bax and Bcl2 protein expression ratio indicated that intrinsic apoptotic pathway may be involved in DS/Cu-induced apoptosis, and this may be caused by simultaneous induction of ROS and inhibition of NF-kB (Yamamoto, et al., 2011).

4.5 Novel cytotoxic compounds for CSCs through the inhibition of NF-kB pathway and its effectors

Actually series of compounds have been tested as inhibitors of Cancer Stem Cells growth and their potent cytotoxic effects on these cells. Exploring the mechanism of action, most of these compounds target the NF-kB pathway or some of the genes regulated by the transcription factor.

CDF (difluorinated-curcumin), a novel analog of the dietary ingredient of curcumin, was examined in combination with 5-fluorouracil and oxaliplatin (5-FU + Ox), the mainstay of colon cancer chemotherapeutic, as a treatment for eliminating colon CSCs. Through multiple and simply methodologies that include real-time RT-PCR, Western blot, MTT assay, caspase-3 activity, colonosphere formation, Hoechst-33342 dye exclusion and NF-κB-ELISA, it was observed that CDF together with 5-FU + Ox were more potent than curcumin in reducing CD44 and CD166 in chemo-resistant colon cancer cells, accompanied by inhibition of growth, induction of apoptosis and disintegration of colonospheres. These changes were associated with down-regulation of the membrane transporter ABCG2 and attenuation of EGFR, IGF-1R, and NF-κB signaling consistent with inactivation of β-catenin, COX-2, c-Myc and Bcl-xL and activation of the pro-apoptotic Bax (Kanwar et al., 2011).

Emerging evidence suggests that highly treatment-resistant tumor-initiating cells (TICs) play a central role in the pathogenesis of pancreatic cancer. Tumor necrosis factor-Related Apoptosis-Inducing Ligand (TRAIL) is considered to be a novel anticancer agent; however, recent studies have shown that many pancreatic cancer cells are resistant to apoptosis induction by TRAIL due to NF-kB signalling. Several chemopreventive agents are able to inhibit NF-kB, for example the broccoli compound sulforaphane. This compound prevents metastasis in clinical studies. Kallifatidis G and coworkers isolated TICs (CD44(+)/CD24(-), CD44(+)/CD24(+) or CD44(+)/CD133(+)) and grew in immunodeficient mice. Specific binding of transcriptionally active cRel-containing NF-kB complexes in TICs was observed. Sulforaphane prevented NF-kB binding, downregulated apoptosis inhibitors and induced apoptosis, together with prevention of clonogenicity. In a xenograft model, sulforaphane strongly blocked tumor growth and angiogenesis, while combination with TRAIL had an additive effect without cytotoxicity in normal cells (Kallifatidis et al., 2009).

5. Conclusions

One of the most important functions in stem cell biology is the regulation of self-renewal. Self-renewal is required by stem cells so that they may last a lifetime, and all stem cells must self-renew and regulate the balance between self-renewal and differentiation. Many pathways that were primarily described in cancer may also regulate normal stem cell development. Among them Oct4 and Nanog, are essential regulators of early development and ES identity. Disruption of either of these factors causes loss of pluripotency. The HMG-box transcription factor, Sox2, heterodimerize with Oct4 in ES cells and regulates expression of Oct4. Each binds to its own promoter and to the promoter of the other two genes. In ES cells Oct4, Sox2 and Nanog act in concert to maintain the pluripotent state. These three transcription factors co-occupy promoters of hundreds of genes, activating some genes and silencing others, in a coordinated fashion, that together promote ES cell self-renewal, however a deregulation of this well orchestrated regulation could generate special conditions that favorites the cancer establishment.

Then there is a very tiny line that differentiates Stem cells and Cancer Stem Cells. However in terms of ill- understanding process our conception of cancer, through the cancer stem cells theory, is changing very fast. The acquisition of stemness like phenotype seems to be involved in several steps of carcinogenesis, then the knowledge generated behind this phenotype could benefits several areas from cell biology to clinical application. Promotion of survival and drug resistance, are the most relevant aspects for a clinical treatment succeed. Gaining a better insight into the mechanisms of stem cell resistance to chemotherapy and the develop of new therapeutic strategies at the molecular level will lead to an effective treatment strategy for preventing the emergence of chemo-resistant cancer cells by eliminating CSCs.

6. References

Akao, Y., Nakagawa, Y., & Naoe, T. (2006). let-7 microRNA functions as a potential growth suppressor in human colon cancer cells. *Biol Pharm Bull*, Vol. 29, pp. 903–906

Alberts, B., Bray, D., Lewis, J., Raff, M., Roberts, K., & Watson, J. (1994). *Molecular biology of the cell.*(3rd ed), Garland Publishing, ISBN 978-0815341055, New York, USA

Al-Hajj, M, Wicha, MS, Benito-Hernandez, A, Morrison, SJ, & Clarke, MF. (2003). Prospective identification of tumorigenic breast cancer cells. *Proc. Natl. Acad. Sci. USA,*Vol. 100, pp.3983-3988

Ali, S. & Coombes, R. (2002). Endocrine-responsive breast cancer and strategies for combating resistance. *Nature Review Cancer,* Vol. 2, pp. 101–112

An, Y., & Ongkeko, W. (2009). ABCG2: the key to chemoresistance in cancer stem cells? *Expert. Opin. Drug Metab. Toxicol.,* Vol. 5, No. 12, pp. 1529-1542

Bar, M., Wyman, S.K., Fritz, B.R., Qi, J., Garg, K.S., Parkin, R.K., et al. (2008). MicroRNA discovery and profiling in human embryonic stem cells by deep sequencing of small RNA libraries. *Stem Cells*, Vol. 26, pp.2496–2505

Boiani, M., Eckardt, S., Scholer, H., & Mc Laughlin, K. (2002). Oct4 distribution and level in mouse clones: consequences for pluripotency. *Genes Dev.*, Vol. 16, pp. 1209—1219

Bonnet, D, & Dick, JE. (1997) Human acute myeloid leukemia is organized as a hierarchy that originates from a primitive hematopoietic cell. *Nat Med,* Vol. 3, pp. 730-737

Braun, S., Vogl, F.D., Naume, B., Janni, W., Osborne, M.P. et al., (2005). A pooled analysis of bonemarrowmicrometastasis in breast cancer. *N. Engl. J. Med.* Vol. 353, pp. 793-802

Bruce, WR, & Van der Gaag, H. (1963). A quantitative assay for the number of murine lymphoma cells capable of proliferation in vivo. *Nature.* Vol. 199, pp. 79-80

Burger, H., Van Tol, H., Boersma, A., Brok, M., Wiemer, E., & Stoter, G. (2004). Imatinib mesylate (STI571) is a substrate for the breast cancer resistance protein (BCRP)/ABCG2 drug pump. *Blood,* Vol. 104, No.9, pp. 2940–2942

Calabrese, J.M., Seila, A.C., Yeo, G.W., & Sharp, P.A.(2007). RNA sequence analysis defines Dicer's role in mouse embryonic stem cells. *Proc Natl Acad Sci USA,* Vol. 104, pp.18097–18102

Calin, G.A., Sevignani, C., Dumitru, C.D., Hyslop, T., Noch, E., Yendamuri, S., et al. (2004). Human microRNA genes are frequently located at fragile sites and genomic regions involved in cancers. *Proc Natl Acad Sci USA*, Vol. 101, pp. 2999–23004

Campioni, N., Pasquali Lasagni, R., Vitucci, C., Filippeti, M., Spagnoli, A., et al., (1986). Peritoneovenous shunt and neoplstic ascites: a 5 years experience report. *J Surg Oncol.* Vol. 33, pp. 31-35

Cavaleri & Schöler, (2009). Molecular basis of pluripotency, In: *Stem Cell Anthology,* B.M. Carlson (Ed), 119-140, Academic press, ISBN 9780123756824, San Diego, USA

Chambers, I., Colby, D., Robertson, M., Nichols, J., Lee, S., Tweedie, S., & Smith, A. (2003). Functional expression cloning of Nanog, a pluripotency sustaining factor in embryonic stem cells. *Cell,* Vol. 113, No 5, pp, 643–655

Cho, R. W., Wang, X., Diehn, M., Shedden, K., Chen, G. Y., et al.,(2008). Isolation and molecular characterization of cancer stem cells in MMTV-Wnt-1 murine breast tumors. *Stem Cells,* Vol. 26, pp. 364-371

Charbod, P. (2010). Bone marrow mesenchymal stem cells: historical overview and concepts. *Human Gene Theraphy,* Vol. 21, No 9, pp 1045-1056

Chen, L., & Liu, L. (2009). Current progress and prospects of induced pluripotent stem cells. *Sci China C Life Sci,*. Vol. 52, No. 7, pp. 622-623

Chiou, S.H., Yu, C.C., Huang, C.Y., Lin, S.C., Liu, C.J., Tsai, T.H.,Chou, S.H.,& Chien, C.S. (2008). Positive Correlations of Oct-4 and Nanog in Oral Cancer Stem-Like Cells and High-Grade Oral Squamous Cell Carcinoma. *Clin Cancer Res.,* Vol. 14, pp. 4085-4095

Cooray, H., Blackmore, C., Maskell, L., & Barrand, M. (2002). Localisation of breast cancer resistance protein in microvessel endothelium of human brain. *Neuroreport,* Vol. 13, No. 16, pp. 2059-2063

Darnell, J. E. Jr. (2002). Transcription factors as targets for cancer therapy. Nature Reviews. Cancer, 2, 740–749

Darnell, J. E. (2005). Validating Stat3 in cancer therapy. Natural Medicines, 11, 595–596

de Sousa, E., Vermeulen, L., Richel, D., & Medema, J. (2011). Targeting Wnt signaling in colon cancer stem cells. *Clin. Cancer Res.,* Vol.15, No. 17, Issue 4, pp. 647-53

Diaz, L.K., Willey, E.L.L. & Venta, L.A. (1999). Are malignant cells displaced by large-gauge needle core biopsy of the breast? *AJR Am. J. Roent Genol.*Vol. 173, pp.1303-1313

D'Ippolito, G., Diabira, S., Howard, G.A., Menei, P., Roos, B.A, & Schiller, P.C. (2004). Marrow-isolated adult multilineage inducible (MIAMI) cells, a unique population of postnatal young and old human cells with extensive expansion and differentiation potential. *J. Cell Sci.* Vol. 117, pp. 2971-2981

Donnenberg, V.S., & Donnenberg, A.D. (2005). Multiple drug resistance in cancer revisited: the cancer stem cell hypothesis. *J. Clin. Pharmacol.* Vol. 45, pp. 872 - 877

Dreesen, O., & Brivanlou, A.H. (2007). Signaling pathways in cancer and embryonic stem cells. *Stem Cell Rev,* Vol. 3, No 1, pp. 7–17

Duesberg, P. (2005). Does aneuploidy or mutation start cancer? *Science,* Vol.307, pp.41-42

Dylla, S.J., Beviglia, L., Park, I.K., Chartier, C., Raval, J., Ngan, L., et al., (2008). Colorectal cancer stem cells are enriched in xenogeneic tumors following chemoteraphy. *PLos ONE,* Vol. 3, pp. e2428

Eriksson, O., Hagmar, B. & Ryd, W. (1984). Effects of fine-needle aspiration and other biopsy procedures on tumor dissemination in mice. *Cancer,* Vol. 54, pp. 73-78

Evans, M., & Kaufman M. (1981). Establishment in culture of pluripotential cells from mouse embryos. *Nature,* Vol. 292, pp. 154–156

Fialkow, P.J.(1972). Use of genetic markers to study cellular origin and development of tumors in human females. *Adv. Cancer Res.*Vol.5, pp.191-226

Fialkow, P.J., Jacobson, R.J. & Papayannopoulou, T. (1977). Chronic myelocytic leukemia: clonal origin in a stem cell common to the granulocyte, erythrocyte, platelet, and monocyte/macrophage. *Am. J. Med.* Vol. 63, pp.125-130

Galli, R., Binda, E., Orfanelli, U, Cipelletti, B., Gritti, A., et al., (2004). Isolation and characterization of tumorigenic, stem-like neural precursors from human glioblastoma.*Cancer Res.*Vol. 64, pp.7011-7021

Garattini, S. (2007). Pharmacokinetics in cancer chemotherapy. *Eur. J. Cancer,* Vol. 43, pp. 271- 282

George, A.A., Franklin, J., Kerkof, K., Shah, A.J., Price, M., et al.,(2001). Detection of leukemic cells in the $CD34^+CD38^-$ bone marrow progenitor population in children with acute lymphoblastic leukemia. *Blood,*Vol. 97, pp. 3925-3930

Ghosh, S., & Karin, M. (2002). Missing pieces in the NF-kB puzzle. *Cell,* Vol 109, pp.81-96

Gilmore, T., Starczynowski, D., Kalaitzidis, D. (2004). RELevant gene amplification in B-cell lymphomas? *Blood,* Vol. 103, pp. 3243–3244.

Goodman, L., Wintrobe, M., Dameshek, W., Goodman, M.J., Gilman, A., & Mc Lennan M. (1946). Nitrogen mustard therapy. *JAMA,* Vol.132, pp. 126– 132

Gorre, M., Mohammed, M., Ellwood, K., Hsu, N., Paquette, R., Rao, P., & Sawyers, C. (2001). Clinical resistance to STI-571 cancer therapy caused by BCR-ABL gene mutation or amplification. *Science,* Vol. 293, pp. 876 - 880

Gottesman, M., Fojo, T., & Bates, S. (2002). Multidrug resistance in cancer: role of ATP-dependent transporters. *Nat. Rev. Cancer,* Vol. 2, pp. 48 - 58

Gottesman, M., Ludwig, J., Xia, D., & Szakacs, G. (2006). Defeating drug resistance in cancer. *Discov Med.,* Vol. 6, No. 31, pp.18–23

Graham, S., Jorgensen, H., & Allan, E. (2002). Primitive, quiescent, Philadelphia-positive stem cells from patients with chronic myeloid leukemia are insensitive to STI571 in vitro. *Blood,* Vol. 99, No.1, pp. 319-325

Hamburger, A.W., & Salmon, S.E. (1977). Primary bioassay of human tumor stem cells. *Science,*Vol. 197, pp. 506-513

Hanahan, D., & Weinberg, R.A. (2000). The hallmarks of cancer. *Cell,* Vol. 100, pp. 57-70

Hanahan, D., & Weinberg, R.A. (2011). Hallmarks of cancer: the next generation. *Cell,* Vol. 144, pp. 646-674.

Hartwell, K.A., Muir, B., Reinhardt, F., Carpenter, A.E., Sgroi, D.C., & Weinberg, R. A. (2006). The Spemann organizer gene, Goosecoid, promotes tumor metastasis. *Proc. Natl. Acad. Sci. U.S.A.,*Vol. 103, pp. 18969–18974

He, L., He, X., Lim, L.P., de Stanchina, E., Xuan, Z., Liang, Y., et al., (2007). A microRNA component of the p53 tumour suppressor network. *Nature,* Vol. 447, pp.1130–1134

Hennessy, B. T., Smith, D. L., Ram, P. T., Lu, Y., & Mills, G. B. (2005). Exploiting the PI3K/AKT pathway for cancer drug discovery. *Nature Reviews Drug Discovery,* Vol. 4, pp. 988–1004

Hill, R.P. & Milas, L. (1989).The proportion of stem cells in murine tumors. *Int. J. Radiat. Oncol. Biol. Phys.* Vol.16, pp.513-518

Hochhaus, A., Kreil, S., Corbin, A., La Rosee, P., Muller, M., Lahaye, T., Hanfstein, B., Schoch, C., Cross, N., Berger, U., Gschaidmeier, H., Druker, B., & Hehlmann, R. (2002). Molecular and chromosomal mechanisms of resistance to imatinib (STI571) therapy. *Leukemia,* Vol. 16, pp. 2190 - 2196

Hombach-Klonisch, S., Paranjothy, T., Wiechec, E., Pocar, P., Mustafa, T., & Seifert, A. (2008). Cancer stem cells as targets for cancer therapy: selected cancers as examples. *Arch. Immunol. Ther. Exp. (Warsz),* Vol. 56, No. 3, pp.165–180

Houghton, P., Germain, G., Harwood, F., Schuetz, J., Stewart, C., & Buchdunger, E. (2004). Imatinib mesylate is a potent inhibitor of the ABCG2 (BCRP) transporter and reverses resistance to topotecan and SN-38 in vitro. *Cancer Res.,* Vol. 64, No.7, pp. 2333–2337

Jamieson, C.H., Ailles, L.E., Dylla, S.J., Muijtjens, & M, Jones C. (2004). Granulocyte-macrophage progenitors as candidate leukemic stem cells in blast-crisis CML. *N Engl. J. Med.* Vol. 351, pp. 657-667

Jiang, Y., Jahagirdar, B.N., Reinhard, R.L., Schwartz, R.E., Keene, C.D., et al., (2002). Pluripotency of mesenchymal stem cells derived from adult marrow. *Nature,* Vol. 418, pp. 41-49

Jordan, C., & Lemishka, I. (1990). Clonal and systemic analysis of long-term hematopoiesis in the mouse. *Genes Dev.,* Vol. 4, pp. 1407–1413

Jorgensen, H. & Holyoake, T. (2011). Characterization of cancer stem cells in chronic myeloid leukaemia. *Int. J. Hematol.,* Vol.93, No. 3, pp. 294-300

Kamel-Reid, S., & Dick, J. (1988). Engraftment of immune-deficient mice with human hematopoietic stem cells. *Science,* Vol. 242, pp. 1706–1709

Kanwar, S.S., Yu,Y., Nautiyal, J., *et al., (2011). Difluorinated-curcumin (CDF): a novel curcumin analog is a potent inhibitor of colon cancer stem-like cells. Pharm Res. Vol. 28, No 4, pp. 827-838]*

Karin, M., & Ben-Neriah, Y. (2000). Phosphorilation meets ubiquitanition:the control of NF-kB activity. *Annu. Rev. Imminol.,* Vol. 18, pp. 621-663

Katoh, M, (2007). Dysregulation of stem cell signaling network due to germline mutation, SNP, Helicobacter pylori infection, epigenetic change and genetic alteration in Gastric cancer. *Cancer Biology and Therapy,* Vol. 6, pp. 832-839

Kelly,P.N., Dakic, A., Adams, J.M., Nutt, S.L. & Strasser, A. (2007).Tumor growth need to not be driven by rare cancer stem cells. *Science,* Vol. 317, pp. 337

Kennedy, J.A., Barabe, F., Poeppl, A.G., Wang, J.C., & Dick, J.E. (2007). Comment on Tumor growth need to not be driven by rare cancer stem cells. Science, Vol. 318, pp.1722; author reply 1722.

Kim, M., Turnquist, H., & Jackson, J. (2002). The multidrug resistance transporter ABCG2 (breast cancer resistance protein 1) effluxes Hoechst 33342 and is over expressed in hematopoietic stem cells. *Clin. Cancer Res.,* Vol.8, No.1, pp. 22-28

Kolligs, F.T., Hu, G, Dang, C.V., & Fearon, E.R. (1999). Neoplastic transformation of RK3E by mutant β-catenin requires deregulation of Tcf/Lef transcription but not activation of c-myc expression. *Mol.Cell. Biol,* Vol. 19, pp. 5696-5706

Langenfeld, E. M., Calvano, S. E., Abou-Nukta, F., Lowry, S. F., Amenta, P., & Langenfeld, J. (2003).The mature bone morphogenetic protein-2 is aberrantly expressed in non-small cell lung carcinomas and stimulates tumor growth of A549 cells. *Carcinogenesis,* Vol. 24, pp. 1445–1454

Langenfeld, E. M., Kong, Y., & Langenfeld, J. (2006). Bone morphogenetic protein 2 stimulation of tumor growth involves the activation of Smad-1/5. *Oncogene,* Vol. 25, pp. 685–692

Lapham, A., Adams, J.E., Paterson, A., Lee, M., Brinmell, M.,& Packham, G. (2009).The Bcl-w promoter is activated by b-catenin/TCF4 in human colorectal carcinoma cells. *Gene*, Vol. 432, No 1-2, pp. 112-117

Leizer, A., Alvero, A., & Fu, H. (2011). Regulation of inflammation by the NF-κB pathway in ovarian cancer stem cells. *Am. J. Reprod. Immunol.*, Vol. 65, No. 4, pp. 438-447.

Leonard, G., Fojo, T., & Bates, S. (2003). The role of ABC transporters in clinical practice. *Oncologist*, Vol. 8, No.5, pp. 411-424

Lin, W., & Karin, M. (2007). A cytokine-mediated link between innate immunity, inflammation and cancer. J. Clin.Invest., Vol. 117, pp. 1175-1183

Lin, T., Chao, C., Saito, S., Mazur, S.J., Murphy, M.E., Appella, E., & Xu, Y. (2005). p53 induces differentiation of mouse embryonic stem cells by suppressing Nanog expression". *Nat. Cell Biol.*, Vol. 7, No 2, pp.165-171

Lobo, N.A., Shimono, Y., Qian, D., & Clarke, M.F. (2007). The biology of cancer stem cells. *Annu. Rev. Cell Dev. Biol.* Vol 23, pp. 675-699

Loeb, L.A. & Harris, C. (2008). Advances in chemical carcinogenesis: A historical review and prospective. *Cancer Res.*, Vol 68, pp. 6863-6872

Masui, H., Nakatake, Y., Toyooka, Y., Shimosato, D., Yagi, R., Takahashi, K., Okochi, H., Okuda, A. et al. (2007). Pluripotency governed by Sox2 via regulation of Oct3/4 expression in mouse embryonic stem cells. *Nature Cell Biology*, Vol. 9, No 6, pp. 625-635

Matsuda, T., Nakamura, T., Nakao, K., Arai, T., Katsuki, M., Heike, T., & Yokota, T. (1999). STAT3 activation is sufficient to maintain an undifferentiated state of mouse embryonic stem cells. EMBO J. Vol. 181, No 15, pp. 4261-4269

Mauro, M.J. & Druker, B.J.(2001). STI571: a gene product-targeted therapy for leukemia. Curr. Oncol. Rep. Vol 3, No 3, pp. 23-227

Mayani, H., Dragowska, W., & Lansdorp, P. (1993). Lineage commitment in human hemopoiesis involves asymmetric cell division of multipotent progenitors and does not appear to be influenced by cytokines. *J Cell Physiol.*, Vol. 157, pp. 579–586

Mayani, H. (2003). A Glance into somatic Stem Cell Biology: Basic Principles, New Concepts and Clinical Relevance. *Archives of Medical Research.*, Vol. 3, pp. 3-15

Melo, J., & Barnes, D. (2007) Chronic myeloid leukaemia as a model of disease evolution in human cancer. *Nat. Rev. Cancer*, Vol.7, pp. 441–453

Mineno, J., Okamoto, S., Ando, T., Sato, M., Chono, H., Izu, H., et al.(2006). The expression profile of microRNAs in mouse embryos. *Nucleic Acids Res*, Vol. 34, pp.1765–1771

Mintz, B., & Illmensee, K. (1975). Normal genetically mosaic mice produced from malignant teratocarcinoma cells. *Proc. Natl. Acad. Sci. USA*, Vol. 72, pp. 3585-3589

Mitsui, K., Tokuzawa, Y., Itoh, H., Segawa, K., Murakami, M., Takahashi, K., Maruyama, M., Maeda, M., & Yamanaka, S. (2003). The homeoprotein Nanog is required for maintenance of pluripotency in mouse epiblast and ES cells. *Cell* , Vol. 113, No 5, pp. 631–642

Miyamoto, T., Weissman, I.L., & Akashi, K. (2000). AML1/ETO-expressing nonleukemic stem cells in acute myelogenous leukemia with 8;21 chromosomal translocation. *Proc. Natl. Acad. Sci. USA*, Vol. 97, pp. 7521-7526

NeRabindran, S., He, H., Singh, M. (1998). Reversal of a novel multidrug resistance mechanism in human colon carcinoma by fumitremorgin C. *Cancer Res.*Vol. 58, No 24, pp. 5850-5858

Nilsson, S., Johnston, H., & Coverdale, J. (2001). Spatial localization of transplanted hemopoietic stem cells: inferences for the localization of stem cell niches. *Blood,* Vol. 97, pp. 2293–2299

Oh, I., & Kwon, K. (2010). Concise review: multiple niches for hematopoietic stem cell regulations. *Stem Cells,* Vol. 28, No. 7, pp. 1243-1249

Orford, K., & Scadden, D. (2008). Deconstructing stem cell self-renewal: genetic insights into cell-cycle regulation. *Nat Rev Genet,* Vol. 9, pp. 115–128

Park, C.H., Bergsagel, D.E., & McCulloch, E.A. (1971). Mouse myeloma tumor stem cells: a primary cell culture assay. *J. Natl. Cancer Inst.* Vol. 46, pp. 411-422

Peter, M.E. (2009). Let-7 and miR-200 MicroRNAs: Guardians against pluripotency and cancer progression. *Cell Cycle,* Vol. 8, No 6, pp. 843–852

Pierce, G.B. & Wallace, C. (1971). Differentiation of malignant to benign cells. *Cancer Res.* Vol 31, pp. 127-134

Piscaglia, A.C., Shupe, T.D., Petersen, B.E., & Gasbarrini, A. (2007). Stem cells, cancer, liver, and liver cancer stem cells: finding a way out of the labyrinth. *Curr. Cancer Drug Targets,* Vol.7, No. 6, pp. 582-590

Pratt, M., Tibbo, E., Robertson, S. (2009). The canonical NF-kappaB pathway is required for formation of luminal mammary neoplasias and is activated in the mammary progenitor population. *Oncogene,* Vol. 30, No. 28, Issue, 30, pp. 2710-2722

Radtke, F., & Raj, K. (2003). The role of Notch in tumorigenesis. Oncogene or tumor suppressor?. *Nat. Rev Cancer.* Vol. 3, pp.765-767

Reguart, N., He, B., Taron, M, You, L, Jablons, D.M., & Rosell, R. (2005). The role of WNT signaling in cancer and stem cells. *Fut Oncol* 1:787-79

Resnick, J., Bixler, L., Cheng, L., & Donovan, P. (1992). Long-term proliferation of mouse primordial germ cells in culture. *Nature,* Vol. 359, pp. 550–551

Reuther, J.,Y., Reuther, G.,W., Cortez, D., Pendergast, A., & Baldwin, A. Jr. (1998). A requirement for NF-kappaB activation in Bcr-Abl-mediated transformation. *Genes Dev.,* Vol. 12, pp. 968–981

Reya, T., Duncan, A.W., Ailles, L., Domen, J., Scherer, D.C., et al., (2003). A role for Wnt signaling in self-renewal of haematopoietic stem cells. *Nature.* Vol. 423, pp. 409-414

Reya, T., Morrison, S., Clarke, M., & Weissman, I. (2001). Stem cells, cancer, and cancer stem cells. *Nature,* Vol. 414, No. 6859, pp. 105–11

Riethdorf, S., Wikman, H., & Pantel, K. (2008). Review: biological relevance of disseminated tumor cells in cancer patients. *Int. J. Cancer,* Vol. 123, pp. 1991-2006

Robey, R., Steadman, K., Polgar, O., et al. (2004). Pheophorbide a is a specific probe for ABCG2 function and inhibition. *Cancer Res.,* Vol. 64, No. 4, pp. 1242-1246

Robey, R., Polgar, O., Deeken, J., et al. (2007). ABCG2: determining its relevance in clinical drug resistance. *Cancer Metastasis Rev.,* Vol.26, No.1, pp. 39-57

Rodriguez-Pinilla, S.M., Sarrio, D., Moreno-Bueno, G., Rodríguez-Gil, Y., Martinez, M.A., Hernandez, L., Hardisson, D., Reis-Filho, J., & Placios, J. (2007). Sox2: a possible driver of the basal-like phenotype in sporadic breast cancer. *Modern Pathology,* Vol. 20, pp. 474–481

Rohwedel, J., Sehlmeyer, U., Shan, J., Meister, A., & Wobus, A. (1996). Primordial germ cell-derived mouse embryonic germ (EG) cells in vitro resemble undifferentiated stem cells with respect to differentiation capacity and cell cycle distribution. *Cell Biol. Int. Rep.* Vol. 20, pp. 579-587

Rosner, M., Vigano, M., Ozato, K., Timmons, P., Poirier, F., Rigby, P., & Staudt, L. (1990). A POU-domain transcription factor in early stem cells and germ cells of the mammalian embryo. *Nature,* Vol. 345, pp. 686—692

Ruiz i Altaba, A., Sanchez, P., & Dahmane, N. (2002). Gli and hedgehog in cancer:tumors,embryos and stem cells. *Nat. Rev. Cancer* Vol. 2, pp. 361-372

Ryd, W., Hagmar, B., & Eriksson, O. (1983). Local tumour cell seeding by fine-needle aspiration biopsy. A semiquantitative study. *Acta Phatol. Microbiol. Inmmunol. Scand.* (A). Vol. 91, pp. 17-21

Saigusa, S., Tanaka, K., Toiyama, Y., Yokoe, T., Okugawa, Y., Ioue, Y., Miki, C.,& Kusunoki, M. (2009). Correlation of CD133, OCT4, and SOX2 in Rectal Cancer and Their Association with Distant Recurrence After Chemoradiotherapy Annals of Surgical *Oncology,* Vol. 16, pp.3488-3498

Sanada, Y., Yoshida, K., Ohara, M., Oeda, M., Konishi, K., & Tsutani, Y.(2006). Histopathologic Evaluation of Stepwise Progression of Pancreatic Carcinoma with Immunohistochemical Analysis of Gastric Epithelial Transcription Factor SOX2: Comparison of Expression Patterns between Invasive Components and Cancerous or Nonneoplastic Intraductal Components. *Pancreas,* Vol. 32, pp.164-170

Scholer, H.R., Balling, R., Hatzopoulos, A.K., Suzuki, N., & Gruss, P. (1989). Octamer binding proteins confer transcriptional activity in early mouse embryogenesis. *EMBO J.* Vol. 8, No 9, pp. 2551-2557

Smith, E.H. (1984). The hazards of fine needle aspiration biopsy. *Ultrasound Med.Biol.,* Vol. 10, pp. 629-634

Smith, AG.(2001). Embryo derived stem cells: of mice and mice. *Annu.Rev.Cell Biol.* Vol.17, pp. 435-462

Slamon, D. J., Clark, G. M., Wong, S. G., Levin, W. J., Ullrich, A., & McGuire, W. L. (1987). Human breast cancer: Correlation of relapse and survival with amplification of the HER-2/neu oncogene. Science, Vol. 235, pp. 177–182

Solter, D., & Knowles, B.B. (1978). Monoclonal antibody defining a stage-specific mouse embryonic antigen (S SEA-1). *Proc. Natl. Acad. Sci. USA.* Vol. 75, No 11, pp. 5565-5569

Soussi, T., & Wiman, K. (2007). Shaping genetic alterations in human cancer: the p53 mutation paradigm. *Cancer Cell,* Vol. 12, pp. 303–312

Southam, C.M., Brunschwig, A., Levin, A.G. & Dizon, Q.S. (1966). Effect of leukocytes on transplantability of human cancer. *Cancer,* Vol.19, pp. 1743-1753

Stefani, G., & Slack, F.J. (2008). Small non-coding RNAs in animal development. *Nat Rev Mol Cell Biol,* Vol. 9, pp.219–230

Sutherland, H.J., Lansdorp, P.M., Henkelman, D.H., & Eaves, C.J. (1990). Functional characterization of individual human hematopoietic stem cells cultured at limiting dilution on supportive marrow stromal layers. *Proc Natl Acad Sci USA.* Vol. 87, pp.3584–3590

Szilvassy, S.J. & Hoffman, R. (1995). Enriched hematopoietic stem cells: basic biology and clinical utility. *Biol. Blood Marrow Transplant.* Vol. 1, No1, pp. 3-17

Tai, M., Chang, C., Olson, L., & Trosko J. (2005). Oct4 expression in adult human stem cells: evidence in support of the stem cell theory of carcinogenesis. *Carcinogenesis,* Vol. 26, No. 2, pp. 495—502

Takahashi, K., & Yamanaka, S. (2006). Induction of pluripotent stem cells from mouse embryonic and adult fibroblast cultures by defined factors. *Cell,* Vol. 126, No. 4, pp. 663-676

Tang, S.N., Junsheng, F., Dara, N., Rodova, M., Shankar, S., & Srivastava, R.K. (2011) Inhibition of sonic hedgehog pathway and plurypotency maintaining factors regulate human pancreatic cancer stem cell characteristics. *Int J. of Cancer.* doi: 10.1002/ijc.26323. Epub ahead of print

Tarin, D., Price, J.E., Kettlewell, M.G., Souter, R.G., Vass, A.C.& Crossley, B. (1984). Clinocopathological observations on metastasis in man studies in patients treated with peritoneovenous shunts. *Br. Med. J.* Vol. 288, pp. 749-751

Thomson, J.A., Itskovitz-Eldor, J., Shapiro, S.S., Waknitz, M., Swiergiel, J.J., Marshall, V.S., Jones, J.M. (1998). Embryonic stem cell lines derived from human blastocyts. *Science,* Vol. 282, pp. 1145-1147

Thomas, T., Miller, C., & Eaves, C. (1999). Purification of hematopoietic stem cells for further biological study. *Methods,* Vol. 17, pp. 202–218

Till, J., & Mc Culloch, E. (1961). A direct measurement of the radiationsensitivity of normal mouse bone marrow cells. *Radiat Res,* Vol. 14, pp. 213–222

Traver, D., Akashi, K., Weissman, I.L., & Lagasse, E. (1998). Mice defective in two apoptosis pathways in the myeloid liunage develop acute myeloblastic leukemia. *Immunity,* Vol. 9, pp. 47-57

Trosko, J., Chang, C., Upham, B., & Tai, M. (2004). Ignored hallmarks of carcinogenesis: stem cells and cell-cell communication. *Ann NY Acad Sci.,* Vol. 1028, pp. 192-201

Trosko, J. (2009). Cancer Stem Cells and Cancer Non stem Cells: From Adult Stem Cells or from Reprogramming of Differentiated Somatic Cells. *Vet. Pathol.,* Vol. 46, pp. 176

Vivanco, I., & Sawyers, C. L. (2002). The phosphatidylinositol 3-Kinase AKT pathway in human cancer. *Nature Reviews. Cancer,* Vol. 2, pp.489–501

Williams, R. (1988). Myeloid leukemia inhibitory factor maintains the developmental potential of embryonic stem cells. *Nature,* Vol. 336, pp. 685–687

Wobus, A., Wallukat, G., & Hescheler, J. (1991). Pluripotent mouse embryonic stem cells are able to differentiate into cardiomyocytes expressing chronotropic responses to adrenergic and cholinergicagents and Ca2? channel blockers. *Differentiation,* Vol. 48, pp. 173–182

Wobus, A. (2010). The Janus face of pluripotent stem cells. Connection between pluripotency and tumourigenicity. *Bioessays,* Vol. 32, pp. 993–1002

Wodinsky, I., Swiniarski, J. & Kensler, C.J. (1967). Spleen colony studies of leukemia L1210. Growth kinetics of lymphocytic L1210 cells in vivo as determined by spleen colony assay. *Cancer Chemother. Rep.* Vol.51, pp. 415-421

Wu, C., & Alman, B. (2008). Side population cells in human cancers. *Cancer Lett.,* Vol. 268, No. 1, pp. 1-9

Yang, J., Mani, S. A., Donaher, J. L., Ramaswamy, S., Itzykson, R. A., Come, C., et al. (2004). Twist, a master regulator of morphogenesis, plays an essential role in tumor metastasis. Cell, 117, 927–939.-51].

Yamamoto, M., Ito, T., & Shimizu, T. (2010). Epigenetic alteration of the NF-κB-inducing kinase (NIK) gene is involved in enhanced NIK expression in basal-like breast cancer. *Cancer Sci.,* Vol. 101, No 11, pp. 2391-2397

Zaehres, H., Lensch, M.W., Daheron, L., Stewart, S.A., Itskovitz-Eldor, J., & Daley, G.Q. (2005). High-efficiency RNA interference in human embryonic stem cells. *Stem Cells,* Vol. 23, No 3, pp. 299–305

Zavadil, J., & Bottinger, E. P. (2005). TGF-beta and epithelial-tomesenchymal transitions. Oncogene, 24, 5764–5774.

Zhang, L., Huang, J., Yang, N., Greshock, J., Megraw, M.S., Giannakakis, A., et al. (2006). microRNAs exhibit high frequency genomic alterations in human cancer. *Proc Natl Acad Sci USA*, Vol. 103, pp.9136–9141

Section 2

Environmental Carcinogenesis

2

Genotoxic Effects of Exposure to Formaldehyde in Two Different Occupational Settings

Susana Viegas[1,2], Carina Ladeira[1,2], Mário Gomes[1], Carla Nunes[2], Miguel Brito[1] and João Prista[2]

[1]*Escola Superior de Tecnologia da Saúde de Lisboa, Instituto Politécnico de Lisboa,*
[2]*Centro de Investigação e Estudos em Saúde Pública, Escola Nacional de Saúde Pública, Universidade Nova de Lisboa, Portugal*

1. Introduction

Formaldehyde (CH_2O), the most simple and reactive aldehyde, is a colorless, reactive and readily polymerizing gas at room temperature (National Toxicology Program [NTP], 2005). It has a pungent suffocating odor that is recognized by most human subjects at concentrations below 1 ppm (International Agency for Research on Cancer [IARC], 2006).

Aleksandr Butlerov synthesized the chemical in 1859, but it was August Wilhelm von Hofmann who identified it as the product formed from passing methanol and air over a heated platinum spiral in 1867. This method is still the basis for the industrial production of formaldehyde today, in which methanol is oxidized using a metal catalyst. By the early 20th century, with the explosion of knowledge in chemistry and physics, coupled with demands for more innovative synthetic products, the scene was set for the birth of a new material–plastics (Zhang et al., 2009).

According to the Report on Carcinogens, formaldehyde ranks 25th in the overall U.S. chemical production, with more than 5 million tons produced each year (NTP, 2005). Formaldehyde annual production rises up to 21 million tons worldwide and it has increased in China with 7.5 million tons produced in 2007. Given its economic importance and widespread use, many people are exposed to formaldehyde environmentally and/or occupationally (Nazaroff et al., 2006).

Commercially, formaldehyde is manufactured as an aqueous solution called formalin, usually containing 37% by weight of dissolved formaldehyde.

This chemical is present in all regions of the atmosphere arising from the oxidation of biogenic and anthropogenic hydrocarbons (International Programme on Chemical Safety [IPCS] 1991; Granby et al., 1997). Formaldehyde concentration levels range typically from 2 to 45 ppbV (parts per billion in a given volume) in urban settings that are mainly governed by primary emissions and secondary formation (Chen et al., 2002; Naya & Nakanishi, 2005).

Primary formaldehyde is emitted from motor vehicles and fugitive industrial emissions, while secondary formaldehyde is produced by the photochemical oxidation of volatile organic compounds (VOCs) as the result of intense sunlight, especially during summer months (Odabasi & Seyfioglu, 2005). In addition, it has been postulated that formaldehyde can be produced by reactions involving anthropogenic and naturally occurring alkenes (Chen et al., 2002).

Removal of formaldehyde from the atmosphere can occur by chemical transformations, rain and snow scavenging of vapours and particles, by dry deposition of particles, and by vapour exchange across the air–water interface. Particle/gas phase distribution of formaldehyde is an important factor in determining its atmospheric fate, transport, and transformation (Odabasi & Seyfioglu, 2005).

Considering indoor air presence, homes containing large amounts of pressed wood products such as hard plywood wall paneling, particleboard, fiberboard, and Urea-Formaldehyde Foam Insulation (UFFI) often have elevated levels of formaldehyde emissions exceeding 0.3 ppm (U. S. Environmental Protection Agency [USEPA], 2007). Since 1985, the Department of Housing and Urban Development has only allowed the use of plywood particleboard that conforms to the 0.4 ppm formaldehyde emission limit in the construction of prefabricated and mobile homes (USEPA, 2007). Formaldehyde emission levels generally decrease as products age. In older homes without UFFI, concentrations of formaldehyde emissions are generally far below 0.1 ppm (USEPA, 2007). This value is close to the indoor limit, 0.1 mg/m^3 (0.08 ppm), recommended by the World Health Organization (World Health Organization - Regional Office of Europe [WHO-ROE], 2006), the limit followed by many other countries including the UK (Committee on the Medical Effects of Air Pollutants [COMEAP], 2004), and China (Standardization Administration of China [SAC], 2002).

Moreover, some studies have reported that seasonal variations resulted in higher indoor formaldehyde concentrations during the summer due to increased off gassing promoted by the higher temperatures (Kinney et al., 2002; Ohura et al., 2006; Yao & Wang., 2005). It seems that besides the type of materials used and home age also the season (warmer temperatures) influence formaldehyde concentrations in indoor settings (Viegas & Prista, 2010; Zhang et al., 2009).

Small amounts of formaldehyde are naturally produced in most organisms, including humans, as a metabolic byproduct (IARC, 2006; NTP, 2005), and are physiologically present in all body fluids, cells and tissues. The endogenous concentration in the blood of humans, monkeys and rats is approximately 2–3 mg/L (0.1 mM) (Casanova et al., 1988; Heck et al., 1985). Formaldehyde is also found in foods, either naturally or as a result of contamination (IARC, 2006). Therefore, everyone is continually exposed to small amounts of formaldehyde, environmentally present in the air, our homes and endogenously in our own bodies (Zhang et al., 2009).

Taking into account occupational settings, exposure involves not only workers in direct production of formaldehyde and products containing it, but also in industries utilizing these products, such as those related with construction and household (Zhang et al., 2009). The most extensive use of formaldehyde is in production of resins with urea, phenol and melamine, and also polyacetal resins. These products are used as adhesives in manufacture of particle-board, plywood, furniture and other wood products (IARC, 2006). Formaldehyde is also used in cosmetics composition and has an important application as a disinfectant and preservative, reason why relevant workplace exposure may also occur in pathology and anatomy laboratories and in mortuaries (Goyer et al., 2004; IARC, 2006; Zhang et al., 2009).

The exposed workers, commonly found in resin production, textiles or other industrial settings, inhale formaldehyde as a gas or absorb the liquid through their skin. Other exposed workers include health-care professionals, medical-lab specialists, morticians and embalmers, all of whom routinely handle bodies or biological specimens preserved with formaldehyde (IARC, 2006; Vincent & Jandel, 2006; Zhang et al., 2009).

Concerning exposure limits in occupational settings, Occupational Safety and Health Administration (OSHA) has established the following standards that have remained the same since 1992: the permissible exposure limit (PEL) is 0.75 ppm (parts per million) in air as an 8-h time-weighted average (TWA_{8h}) and the short-term (15 min) exposure limit (STEL) is 2 ppm. American Conference of Governmental Industrial Hygienists (ACGIH) recommended threshold limit value (TLV) is 0.3 ppm as a ceiling value. The National Institute of Occupational Safety and Health (NIOSH) recommends much lower exposure limits of 0.016 ppm (TWA_{8h}) and 0.1 ppm (STEL), above which individuals are advised to use respirators if working under such conditions. In Portugal, the Portuguese Norm (NP 1796 - 2007) points also 0.3 ppm as a ceiling value.

The primary metabolite of formaldehyde is formate which is not as reactive as formaldehyde itself and can either enter into the one-carbon metabolic pool for incorporation into other cellular components, be excreted as a salt in the urine, or further metabolized to carbon dioxide (Agency for Toxic Substances and Disease Registry [ATSDR], 1999). The metabolic pathway to formate production is catalyzed by cytosolic glutathione (GSH)- dependent formaldehyde dehydrogenase (FDH). The reaction of formaldehyde with GSH yields (S)-hydroxymethylglutathione which, in the presence of NAD+ and FDH, forms the thiol ester of formic acid via the action of (S)-formyl glutathione hydrolase (SFGH) (Pyatt et al., 2008).

There is scientific evidence conclusively demonstrating that inhaled formaldehyde does not enter the systemic circulation to modify normally present endogenous levels (ATSDR, 1999; Heck & Casanova, 2004). This is likely due to the high water solubility of formaldehyde and its rapid metabolism. The lack of systemic distribution is evidenced by a variety of studies in rodents, monkeys and humans (Pyatt et al., 2008).

It seems clear that as long as inhaled levels of formaldehyde are below concentrations that can be rapidly metabolized by tissue formaldehyde dehydrogenase and other highly efficient detoxification enzymes, normal endogenous concentrations (0.1 mM) of formaldehyde in the blood do not increase (ATSDR, 1999; Heck & Casanova, 2004).

Human studies have shown that chronic exposure to formaldehyde by inhalation is associated with eye, nose and throat irritation (Arts et al., 2008). Sensory irritation leads to reflex responses such as sneezing, lacrimation, rhinorrhea, coughing, vasodilatation and changes in the rate and depth of respiration. The latter results are a decrease in the total amount of inhaled material resulting in a protective effect to the individual. Trigeminus stimulation is not necessarily an indication of cell or tissue damage. At higher concentrations formaldehyde will lead to cytotoxic reactions; this cytotoxic respiratory tract irritation is a localized pathophysiological response to a chemical, involving local redness, swelling, or itching (Arts et al., 2006).

Formaldehyde was long considered as a probable human carcinogen (Group 2A chemical) based on experimental animal studies and limited evidence of human carcinogenicity. More recently, several studies report a carcinogenic effect in humans after chronic exposure to formaldehyde, in particular an increased risk for nasopharyngeal cancer (Armstrong et al., 2000; Coggon et al., 2003; Hildesheim et al., 2001; Lubin et al., 2004; Vaughan et al., 2000). Since 2006, IARC classifies formaldehyde as carcinogenic to humans (Group 1), based on sufficient evidence in humans and in experimental animals (IARC, 2006). IARC also concluded that there is a "strong but not sufficient evidence for a causal association between leukemia and occupational exposure to formaldehyde".

The "strong" evidence for a causal relationship between formaldehyde exposure and leukaemia comes from recent updates of two of the three major industrial cohort studies of formaldehyde-exposed workers (Hauptmann et al., 2003; Pinkerton et al., 2004). These data have strengthened a potential causal association between leukemia and occupational exposure to formaldehyde, especially for myeloid leukemia (Zhang et al., 2009).

Nevertheless, some authors have argued that it is biologically implausible for formaldehyde to cause leukaemia (Cole & Axten, 2004; Marsh & Youk, 2004). Their primary arguments against the human leukemogenicity of formaldehyde are: (1) it is unlikely to reach the bone marrow and cause toxicity due to its highly reactive nature; (2) there is no evidence that it can damage the stem and progenitor cells, the target cells for leukemogenesis; and (3) there is no credible experimental animal model for formaldehyde-induced leukaemia. This led Pyatt et al., (2008) to recently comment that "the notion that formaldehyde can cause any lymphohematopoietic malignancy is not supported with either epidemiologic data or current understanding of differing etiologies and risk factors for the various hematopoietic and lymphoproliferative malignancies". Indeed, IARC itself concluded that "based on the data available at this time, it was not possible to identify a mechanism for the induction of myeloid leukaemia in humans" and stated that "this is an area needing more research" (IARC, 2006; Cogliano et al., 2005; Zhang et al., 2009).

However, recently, IARC reaffirmed the classification of formaldehyde in Group I, based on sufficient evidence in humans of nasopharyngeal cancer. Considering the possible association with leukemia the epidemiological evidence has become stronger and IARC has concluded that there is sufficient evidence for leukaemia, particularly myeloid leukaemia (Baan et al., 2009; Hauptmann et al., 2009; IARC, 2006).

Moreover, in 2010 Schwilk and colleagues performed an up-dated meta-analyses focusing in higher exposure groups and myeloid leukemia and included two large recent studies and conclude that formaldehyde exposure is associated with increased risks of leukemia, particularly myeloide leukemia and highlight the importance of focusing on high-exposure groups and myeloid leukemia when evaluating the human carcinogenicity of formaldehyde (Schwilk et al., 2010).

In the case of formaldehyde exposure assessment and considering that health effects seems to be mainly related with the high concentration peaks than with long time exposure at low levels, the strategy to perform exposure assessment in occupational settings must be based on the determination of ceilings concentrations. This option might be the best to evaluate exposures and to obtain data for risk assessment development (Hauptmann et al., 2009; IARC, 2006).

Manifold in vitro studies clearly indicated that formaldehyde can induce genotoxic effects in proliferating cultured mammalian cells (IARC, 2006). Furthermore, some in vivo studies detected changes in epithelial cells (oral and nasal) and in peripheral lymphocytes related to formaldehyde exposure (Speit & Schmid, 2006; Suruda et al., 1993).

Frequency of micronucleus (MN) in buccal and/or nasal mucosa cells is being used to investigate local genotoxicity. According to reports concerning experimental genotoxicity studies, MN are the most sensitive genetic endpoints for detection of formaldehyde induced genotoxicity (Merck & Speit, 1998). Thus, MN test with exfoliated cells could be a powerful tool for detection of local genotoxic effects in humans, which is fundamental for hazard identification and risk estimation (Speit & Schmid, 2006).

MN in peripheral blood lymphocytes has been extensively used to evaluate the presence and extend of chromosome damage in human populations exposed to genotoxic agents. As advantages, this MN test provides a reliable measure of chromosomal breakage and loss at lower cost and more easily than chromosomal aberrations. Moreover, the availability of cytokinesis-block technique eliminates potential background caused by effects on cell division kinetics (Bonassi et al., 2001).

Research work has been developed to know occupational exposure to formaldehyde in two different occupational settings (resins production and in pathology and anatomy laboratories) from Portugal and, also, study eventual health effects related with exposure. The objective of this chapter is to describe the work developed and discuss the obtained results.

2. Research developed

2.1 Materials and methods

2.1.1 Subjects

This study was carried out in Portugal, in 80 workers occupationally exposed to formaldehyde vapours: 30 workers from formaldehyde and formaldehyde-based resins production factory and 50 from 10 pathology and anatomy laboratories. A control group of 85 non-exposed subjects was considered. All subjects were provided with the protocol and with the consent form, which they read and signed.

Health conditions, medical history, medication and lifestyle factors for all studied individuals, as well as information related to working practices (such as years of employment) were obtained through a standard questionnaire.

2.1.2 Exposure assessment

Two different exposure assessment methods were, simultaneously, applied in the 10 anatomy and pathology laboratories in Portuguese hospitals and in the formaldehyde and formaldehyde-based resins production factory, in order to assess formaldehyde occupational exposure. Environmental monitoring was performed between the period of September 2007 and March of 2008.

In these two occupational settings were identified different exposure groups. In laboratories were defined three, namely pathologists, technicians and technical assistant. Also, in the factory were define three groups - production of resins, impregnation and quality control. These definitions were based essentially on activities similarity.

2.1.3 Methods

Method 1

In one of the methods 30 environmental samples were obtained by personal air sampling with low flow rate (0.01 to 0.10 L/min) pumps (Zambelli) during a typical working day. The sorbent tubes used were impregnated with 10% (2-hydroxymethyl)piperidine. Sampling time was 6 to 7 hours. Two to three samples were collected in each laboratory by the use of electric flow pumps which were placed in a worker of each exposure group.

Formaldehyde levels were measured by Gas Chromatography (GC). Capillary column: Supelcowax^{10} - 30 m x 0.32 mm x 0.5 µm; analyte: oxazolidine derivative of formaldehyde; desorption: 1 mL toluene; 60 min ultrasonic; injection volume: 1 µL splitless; split vent time 30 sec; temperature: injector: 250 °C, detector: 300 °C, column: 70 °C for 1 min; 15 °C/min; hold at 240 °C for 10 min; carrier gas: He – 1.5 mL/min; calibration: formalin solution spiked on sorbent – 4.7 µg/mL, 6.0 µg/mL, 13.0 µg/mL, 25.0 µg/mL, 40.0 µg/mL, 50.0 µg/mL, 100.0 µg/mL e 200.0 µg/mL; calibration curve: $y=0.008522x - 0.008109$ $r^2 = 0.999968$, LOD: 1µg/sample . Analysis and time-weighted average (TWA_{8h}) estimated according to the National Institute of Occupational Safety and Health method - NIOSH 2541 (National Institute of Occupational Safety and Health [NIOSH], 1994).

Method 2

Ceiling values for formaldehyde exposure were obtained using Photo Ionization Detection (PID) direct-reading equipment (with an 11.7 eV lamp) designated by First-Check, from Ion Science. This equipment accurately detects formaldehyde from 1 ppb to 10,000 ppm and performs automatically data log readings from the sensor on a second basis. Measurements were performed in each task and readings were stored in instrument internal memory with a date and time stamp. At the same time it was performed video recording and synchronized with real-time exposure data obtained with PID equipment followed by combination of the exposure profile with the video image of worker activity.

With this method it was possible to establish a relation between worker activities and ceiling values, and to determine principal emission sources.

Eighty three activities were studied in the 10 laboratories and three activities in the factory. All tasks were studied in normal conditions, namely using ventilation dispositive and, as usual, none of the workers was using masks to protect from formaldehyde vapours.

In both methods sampling/measures were performed near workers respiratory system.

Data obtained from NIOSH 2451 method was compared with reference value from OSHA (TLV-TWA=0.75 ppm) because there is no reference in Portugal for this exposure metric. The ceiling values obtained from PID method were compared with reference value from Portuguese Norm 1796-2007 (0.3 ppm).

2.1.4 Biological monitoring

To evaluate the effects of the occupational exposure, the study of effect biomarkers was conducted. The biomarkers of effect studied were specifically genotoxicity biomarkers, namely micronuclei in two different biological matrixes - peripheral blood lymphocytes and buccal exfoliated cells.

The protocol used to measure the MN in peripheral blood lymphocytes was the fully validated cytokinesis-blocked micronucleus assay (CBMN), developed by Fenech [20], where it is used citochalasin B to block the cytokinesis in order to lymphocytes had a binucleated appearance. Heparinized blood samples were obtained by venipuncture from all subjects and freshly collected blood was directly used for the MN test. Lymphocytes were isolated using Ficoll-Paque gradient and placed in RPMI 1640 culture medium with L-glutamine and red phenol added with 10% inactivated fetal calf serum, 50 ug/ml streptomycin + 50U/mL penicillin, and 10 ug/mL phytohaemagglutinin. Duplicate cultures from each subject were incubated at 37°C in a humidified 5% CO_2 incubator for 44h, and cytochalasin-b 6 ug/mL was added to the cultures in order to prevent cytokinesis. After 28h incubation, cells were spun onto microscope slides using a cytocentrifuge. Smears were air-dried and double stained with May-Grünwald-Giemsa and mounted with Entellan. The frequencies of binucleated cells with MN were determined analyzing 1000 lymphocytes from two slides for each subject.

The optimal protocol of MN test for buccal exfoliated cells was performed after many experiments. In order to reach the optimal protocol, different techniques of collecting the cells and the staining were done.

Concerning to the sample collection, it was considered that the best way of obtaining the sample it was by scrapping the inner checks of the individuals with an endobrush and directly performed a smear in two slides. The samples were immediately fixed with Mercofix®, a methanol based preservative.

The staining protocols selected were based on the affinity of the stains with the nucleus: Hematoxilin-Eosin, Hematoxilin, Giemsa, May-Grunwald Giemsa, Papanicolaou, Feulgen with Light Green and Feulgen.

The reliable results were achieved with Feulgen without counterstain (Nersesyan et al., 2006). This technique consists in a first step of hydrolysis with HCL 5M followed by washing with distillate water, incubation with Schiff Reagent and tap water final washing. The slides were allowed to air dried, mounted with entellan®. Two thousand cells were scored from each individual. Only cells containing intact nuclei, neither clumped nor overlapping were included in the analysis.

The criteria for scoring the nuclear abnormalities in lymphocytes and MN in buccal cells were described by Fenech et al. (1999) and Tolbert et al. (1991), respectively.

2.2 Results

2.2.1 Characteristics of the studied population

The characterization of the population studied is summarized in Table 1. Controls and exposed workers did not differ significantly in age and in smoking habits. Only for gender distribution a significant difference was found between the two groups (p=0.002), due to the larger number of women in the control group.

	Control Group	Exposed Group	*P* value
Number of subjects	85	80	
Gender			
Male	31 (36.6%)	48 (60.0%)	0.002
Female	54 (63.5%)	32 (40.0%)	
Age (years)			
Range	20-55	19-56	
Mean	33.87	35.74	0.180
St. Deviation	8.262	9.470	0.024
Smoking status			
Non-smokers	59 (69.4%)	55 (68.8%)	0.927
Smokers	26 (30.6%)	25 (31.3%)	
Years of exposure			
Range	------	1 - 35	

Table 1. Characterization of the studied population

None of the individuals presented relevant information about health conditions, medical history, medication and lifestyle factors that could influence the results of MN test.

2.2.2 Exposure assessment

Formaldehyde exposure values were determined using the above described methods: NIOSH 2541 for average concentrations (TWA_{8h}) and PID method to obtain ceiling concentrations (Tables 2 and 3).

Laboratories	Exposure Groups	FA TWA_{8h} n=29 (ppm)	FA Ceiling * n=83 (ppm)	Range Ceiling values (ppm)	Mean Ceiling values (ppm)
A	Technical Assistant	0.27	2.51	1.05 - 2.51	1.78
	Pathologist	<LOD	3.19	0.34 - 3.19	1.04
	Technician	0.16	NM	--------	
B	Technical Assistant	0.15	0.62	0.62	------
	Pathologist	0.24	2.71	1.49 - 3.36	2.23
	Technician	0.16	3.36	1.91 - 3.36	2.31
C	Technical Assistant	0.12	0.53	0.53	-----
	Pathologist	0.47	2.93	1.53 - 2.93	2.18
	Technician	0.51	2.28	2.22 - 2.28	2.25
D	Technical Assistant	< LOD	NM	------	
	Pathologist	0.07	2.31	2.09 - 2.31	2.21
	Technician	0.11	0.85	0.85	------
E	Technical Assistant	< LOD	NM	------	------
	Pathologist	0.06	1.10	0.95 - 1.10	1.03
	Technician	0.07	0.85	0.85	-----
F	Technical Assistant	0.09	NM	------	-----
	Pathologist	0.23	0.34	0.22 - 0.34	0.28
	Technician	0.12	0.28	0.28	-----

Laboratories	Exposure Groups	FA TWA_{8h} n=29 (ppm)	FA Ceiling * n=83 (ppm)	Range Ceiling values (ppm)	Mean Ceiling values (ppm)
G	Technical Assistant	0.16	0.71	0.64 - 1.71	0.67
	Pathologist	0.05	2.81	0.18 - 2.81	0.56
	Technician	0.04	1.26	1.26	-----
H	Technical Assistant	0.25	0.68	0.68	----
	Pathologist	0.11	2.08	1.21 - 2.08	1.65
	Technician	0.25	0.68	0.68	----
I	Technical Assistant	0.05	0.95	0.95	----
	Pathologist	< LOD	0.47	0.21 - 0.47	0.34
	Technician	0.06	NM	----	----
J	Technical Assistant	NM	NM	----	----
	Pathologist	0.13	5.02	1.15 - 5.02	3.24
	Technician	0.08	4.32	4.32	----

* Higher values for each exposure group
< LOD - Below the Detection limit
FA-formaldehyde
NM - Not measured

Table 2. Formaldehyde exposure results in laboratories

Exposure groups	FA TWA_{8h} n=3 (ppm)	FA Ceiling * n=3 (ppm)	Range Ceiling values (ppm)	Mean Ceiling values (ppm)
Production of resins	NM	Collecting a sample of the reactor 1.02	0.01 - 1.02	0.15
Impregnation	< LOD	Operation of impregnation machine 1.04	0.00 - 1.04	0.21
Quality control	< LOD	analyze a resin sample 0.52	0.01 - 0.52	0.08

* Higher values for each exposure group
< LOD - Below the Detection limit
NM - Not measured
FA -formaldehyde

Table 3. Formaldehyde exposure results in the factory

All of the results for time-weighted average concentrations (TWA_{8h}) not exceeded OSHA reference value (0.75 ppm), with the majority of values falling below the method detection limited.

On the opposite, for ceiling concentrations all the higher results obtained for each exposure group in each occupational setting exceeded the reference value (0.3 ppm). In laboratories, values lied between 0.18 ppm and 5.02 ppm, with a mean of 2.52 ppm. In the factory the concentration values registered each second lied between 0.0 and 1.02 ppm.

The three activities studied in the factory have result above the reference value for ceiling concentrations (0.3 ppm).

In production of resins the higher concentration value was obtained during the collection of a sampling in resins reactor performed by a production operator. In this case and during operation of impregnation machine there were not local exhaust ventilation dispositive. Only in the "quality control" exposure group there was a small hotte that is not normally used to perform quality analysis of resins.

In the case of laboratories, all of them had, at least, one task with a higher result than the reference value (0.3 ppm) (Figure 1).

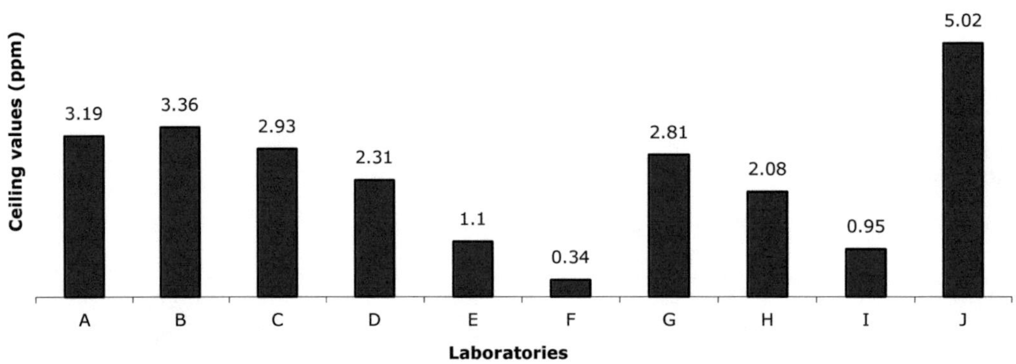

Fig. 1. Higher ceiling value obtained in each laboratory

Considering all of the 83 tasks studied in the laboratories (Table 4), 93% of the results were higher than the reference value for ceiling concentrations (0.3 ppm).

Highest exposure level was observed during "macroscopic examination" of formaldehyde-preserved specimens. This task is developed in a macroscopic bench with local exhaust ventilation. In all the laboratories studied was verified that ventilation was functioning normally.

The task "data registration" showed also a high formaldehyde concentration value, being important to note that this task occurs during macroscopic examination (Table 4).

Concerning the 69 macroscopic examinations, the most frequent task develop in this laboratories, it was possible to verify that near 93% of formaldehyde concentration values were higher than 0.3 ppm.

In this occupational setting, highest score for ceiling values was identified in the results of the exposure group "Pathologists" and the highest mean was obtained for the "Technicians" group (Table 5).

It is important to consider that none of the workers of the two occupational settings were using appropriate respiratory protection during the tasks studied.

Tasks	**Number**	**Ceiling Values (ppm)**	**Exposed Workers**
Macroscopic examination	69	5.02	Pathologist
Disposal of specimen and used solutions	5	0.95	Technicians and Technical Assistant
Jar filling	2	2.51	Technical Assistant
Data registration	3	4.32	Technicians
Specimen wash	2	2.28	Technicians
Biopsy	2	1.91	Technicians

Table 4. Formaldehyde exposure during laboratories tasks

Exposure Groups	**Tasks studied***	**Range** (ppm)	**Mean** (ppm)	**St. Deviation** (ppm)
Technical Assistant	9	0.28 - 2.51	0.86	0.58
Pathologist	65	0.21 - 5.02	1.42	1.07
Technician	14	0.68 - 4.32	2.04	0.95

* some activities involved the simultaneously exposure of two groups

Table 5. Ceiling results for each exposure group

2.2.3 Biological monitoring

Table 6 showed that the frequency of MN in occupationally exposed workers was significantly higher in comparison with the control group, both in peripheral blood lymphocytes ($p<0.001$) and in epithelial buccal cells ($p<0.001$).

	Controls	Exposed		
		Factory	Pathology and anatomy laboratories	Total
MN PBL [1] Mean ± Std. Dev	1.17±1.95	1.76±2.07	3.70±3.86	2.97±3.42
MN EBC[2] Mean ± Std. Dev	0.13±0.48	1.27±1.55	0.64±1.74	0.88±1.69

[1] Peripheral Blood Lymphocytes
[2] Epithelial Buccal Cells

Table 6. Frequency of MN in the studied population

When analyzing each occupational setting separately, we found significant differences in MN frequencies in peripheral blood lymphocytes ($p < 0.001$) and in epithelial buccal cells ($p<0.005$) between the laboratories and control groups. Concerning the factory group, significant differences in MN frequencies were only detected in epithelial buccal cells ($p<0.001$).

Finally, it was compared MN frequencies between the two exposed groups and found that MN frequency in peripheral blood lymphocytes was significantly higher in the laboratories group ($p<0.005$), but respecting to epithelial buccal cells there was no significant difference between them ($p=0.108$).

In what concern to the three exposure groups studied in the pathology anatomy laboratories, the pathologists group has higher MN mean in lymphocytes and the technician had higher MN mean in buccal cells (Table 7).

	Pathology and anatomy laboratories		
	Pathologist	Technician	Technical Assistant
MN PBL Mean ± Std. Error of Mean	5.00±1.24	3.76±0.647	4.13±1.55
MN EBC Mean ± Std. Error of Mean	0.58±0.434	1.18±0.406	0.88±0.611

Table 7. Frequency of MN in the exposure groups of laboratories

Factory results reveal quality control group with higher MN mean in lymphocytes and also in buccal cells (Table 8).

	Factory		
	Resins Production	Impregnation	Quality control
MN PBL Mean ± Std. Error of Mean	1.85±2.48	1.16±1.04	4.5±0.7
MN EBC Mean ± Std. Error of Mean	0.66±0.94	1.75±1.79	3.5±0.5

Table 8. Frequency of MN in the exposure groups of factory

2.3 Discussion

As indicated by several studies (IARC, 2006; Orsière et al., 2006; Shaham et al., 2003) exposure assessment in present investigation demonstrates that both occupational settings studied involve exposure to high peak formaldehyde concentrations.

The importance of this consideration lies in the fact that health effects (cancer) linked to formaldehyde exposure are more related with peaks of high concentrations than with long time exposure at low levels (IARC, 2006; Pyatt et al., 2008). Moreover, the choice of exposure metric should be based on the most biologically relevant exposure measure in order to diminish misclassification of exposure, thus leading to attenuated exposure-response relationships (Preller et al., 2004). Furthermore, high exposures of short duration (peaks) are of special concern, because they can produce an elevated dose rate at target tissues and organs, potentially altering metabolism, overloading protective and repair mechanisms and amplifying tissue responses (Preller et al., 2004; Smith, 2001). In addition, Pyatt et al. (2008) pointed out, as a limitation in most epidemiological studies, the lack of data about exposure to peak concentrations. Therefore, in those studies, health effects resulting from occupational exposure to formaldehyde are associated to exposure exclusively based on time-weighted average concentrations (Pyatt et al., 2008). Until 2004 only two studies concerning the association between exposure to formaldehyde and nasopharyngeal cancer that presented data on exposure to ceiling concentrations obtained higher relative risk values compared with the other studies (Hauptmann et al., 2004; Pinkerton et al., 2004; Zhang et al., 2009).

Recently Hauptmann and colleagues have found that mortality rate from leukemia increased significantly not just with number of years of activity, in this case embalming, but also with increasing peak formaldehyde exposure (Dreyfuss, 2010; Hauptmann et al., 2009).

Results in laboratories indicate "macroscopic examination" as the task involving the highest exposure. This is probably because precision and very good visibility is needed and, therefore, pathologists must lean over the specimen with consequent increase of proximity to formaldehyde emission sources. Studies developed by Goyer et al., (2004) and Orsière et al., (2006) support that proximity to impregnated specimens promotes higher exposure to formaldehyde. "Pathologist" is normally the exposure group that performs this task. However, the "Technician" group obtained, simultaneously, higher TWA_{8h} and higher mean of ceiling values. This can be due to the fact that this is the group envolved in more tasks related with formaldehyde exposure, during the working day.

In the case of the factory, the task "collecting a sample of the reactor" involved a manual process. Probably the proximity and reactor open promote exposure.

It is important to refer that these type of information (exposure determinants, emission sources and exposed workers) was only possible to obtain because video recording could be performed simultaneously with concentration measurements.

This resource gives opportunity to directly relate performance with exposure (Mcglothlin, 2005; Ryan et al., 2003; Rosén et al., 2005). Additionally, real-time measurements are useful also for evaluating engineering controls and their efficacy (Yokel & MacPhail, 2011).

In addition, and in agreement with other studies (Kromouht, 2002; Meijster et al., 2008; Susi & Schneider, 1995), it is possible to conclude that TWA_{8h} measurements give poor information and is of less utility in the identification of tasks that should be targeted for control.

Long exposures to formaldehyde, as those to which some workers are subjected for occupational reasons, are suspected to be associated with genotoxic effects that can be evaluated by biomarkers (Conaway et al., 1996; IARC, 2006; Viegas & Prista, 2007). In this study, the results suggest that workers in pathological anatomy laboratories are exposed to formaldehyde levels that exceed recommended exposure criteria and a statistically significant association was found between formaldehyde exposure and biomarkers of genotoxicity, namely MN in lymphocytes and buccal cells.

Chromosome damage and effects upon lymphocytes arise because formaldehyde escapes from sites of direct contact, such as mouth, originating nuclear alterations in lymphocytes of those exposed (He & Jin, 1998; Orsière et al., 2006; Ye et al., 2005; Zhang et al., 2009).

Our results corroborate previous reports (Ye et al., 2005) that lymphocytes can be compromised by long term exposures. Moreover, the changes in peripheral lymphocytes can be a sign that the cytogenetic effects triggered by formaldehyde can reach tissues faraway from the site of initial contact (Suruda et al., 1993). Long term exposures to high concentrations of formaldehyde indeed appear to have a potential for generalized DNA damage. In experimental studies with animals, local genotoxic effects following formaldehyde exposure have been previously demonstrated to give rise to DNA-protein cross links, structural chromosomal aberrations, and aberrant cells (IARC, 2006). In our research work the MN frequency in peripheral blood lymphocytes was significantly higher in the laboratories group in comparison with the factory, probably because the years of exposure are higher in the first group.

In humans, formaldehyde exposure is associated with an increase in the frequency of MN in buccal epithelium cells (Burgaz et al., 2002; Speit et al., 2007) as corroborated by the results presented here.

Suruda el al. (1993) claims that although changes in oral and nasal epithelial cells and peripheral blood cells do not indicate a direct mechanism leading to carcinogenesis, they do indicate that DNA alterations took place. It thus appears reasonable to conclude that formaldehyde is a risk factor for those that are occupationally exposed in these two occupational settings (IARC, 2006).

In human biomonitoring studies it is important to assess the influence of major confounding factors such as gender, age and smoking habits in the endpoints studied. However, in ours results no significant differences were obtained in MN frequencies between women and men (both in peripheral blood lymphocytes and epithelial buccal cells). However, in other studies an increase in MN frequencies in women was found. Current knowledge on the effect of gender on genetic damage determines a 1.5-fold greater MN frequency in females than in males (Fenech et al., 2003; Wojda et al., 2007), witch can be explained by preferential aneugenic events involving the X-chromossome. Surralés et al. (1996) reported an excessive overrepresentation of this chromosome in micronucleic lymphocytes cultured from women.

Tobacco smoke contains a high number of mutagenic and carcinogenic substances and is causally linked to an elevated incidence of several forms of cancers (IARC, 1985). Hence, smoking is an important variable to consider in biomonitoring studies and, particularly in this study since formaldehyde is present in tobacco smoke (IARC, 2006). The effect of tobacco smoking on MN frequency in human cells has been object of study. In most reports the results were unexpected, as in many instance smokers had lower frequencies of MN than non-smokers (Bonassi et. 2003; Orsière et al., 2006). In the present study no significant differences were found in MN (peripheral blood lymphocytes and epithelial buccal cells) between smokers and non-smokers. These findings are similar to results obtained in the study of Bonassi et al., (2003). These authors recommend that quantitative data about smoking habit should be collected because the sub-group of heavy smokers (≥30 cigarettes per day) can influence the results. For notice, the questionnaire results of this study revealed no heavy smokers in these two workers groups.

3. Conclusion

Some preventive measures can be applied to reduce exposure to formaldehyde in these two occupational settings. In the case of anatomy and pathology laboratories exposure reduction can be achieved by the use of adequate local exhausts ventilation, relocation of the specimen containers to areas with isolated ventilation and using hooded enclosures over such containers.

For the factory, preventive measures must consider automating some processes like sampling in reactors and, additionally, promote the use of the existing located ventilation dispositive.

Exposure assessment methods applied in the research developed permitted to conclude that TWA_{8h} measurements give poor information concerning to preventive measures priority and CBMN assay applied to assess genotoxic effects is a screening technique that can be used for clinical prevention and management of workers under occupational carcinogenic risks, namely exposure to a genotoxic agent such as formaldehyde.

The most recent studies suggest that future research is warranted to more effectively assess the risk of leukemia arising from formaldehyde exposure and to better explain some inconsistencies in mode of action and, also, to understand the role of short-term peak exposures.

4. References

Agency for Toxic Substances and Disease Registry (ATSDR) (1999). Toxicological Profile for Formaldehyde. US Department Of Health And Human Services, Public Health Service.

Armstrong, R., Imrey, P., Lye, M., Armstrong, M., Yu, M. & Sani, S. (2000). Nasopharyngeal carcinoma in Malaysian Chinese: occupational exposures to particles, formaldehyde and heat. *Int J Epidemiol*, 29,991-998.

Arts, J. Rennen, M. & de Heer, C. (2006). Inhaled formaldehyde: evaluation of sensory irritation in relation to carcinogenicity. *Regul. Toxicol. Pharmacol.* 44, 144–160.

Arts, J., Muijser, H., Kuper, C., & Woutersen, R. (2008). Setting an indoor air exposure limit for formaldehyde: Factors of concern. *Regulatory Toxicology and Pharmacology*, 52, 189–194

Baan, R., Grosse, Y., Straif, K., Secretan, B., El Ghissassi, F., Bouvard, V., Benbrahim-Tallaa, L., Guha, N., Freeman, C., Galichet, L. & Cogliano V. (2009). On behalf of the WHO International Agency for Research on Cancer Monograph Working Group, A review of human carcinogens. Part F. Chemical agents and related occupations. *The Lancet Oncol.*, 10, 1143–1144.

Bonassi, S., Fenech, M., Lando, C., Lin, YP., Ceppi, M., Chang, WP., Holland, N., Kirsch-Volders, M., Zeiger, E., Ban, S., Barale, R., Bigatti, MP., Bolognesi, C., Jia, C., Di Giorgio, M., Ferguson, LR., Fucic, A., Lima, OG., Hrelia, P., Krishnaja, AP., Lee, TK., Migliore, L., Mikhalevich, L., Mirkova, E., Mosesso, P., ,Müller, WU., Odagiri, Y., Scarffi, MR., Szabova, E., Vorobtsova, I., Vral, A. & Zijno, A. (2001). Human MicroNucleus Project: international database comparison for results with the cytokinesis-block micronucleus assay in human lymphocytes: I. Effect of laboratory protocol, scoring criteria, and host factors on the frequency of micronuclei. *Environ Mol Mutagen*, 37, 31-45.

Burgaz, S., Erdem, O., Çakmak, G. & Karakaya, A. (2002). Cytogenetic analysis of buccal cells from shoe-workers and pathology and anatomy laboratory workers exposed to n-hexane, toluene, methyl ethyl ketone and formaldehyde. *Biomarkers.*, 2, 151-161.

Chen, J., So, S., Lee, H., Fraser, MP., Curl, R., Harman, T. & Tittel, F. (2004). Atmospheric Formaldehyde Monitoring in the Greater Houston Area in 2002. *Applied Spectroscopy*, 58, 2.

Coggon, D., Harrism EC., Poole, J. & Palmer, KT. (2003). Extended follow-up of a cohort of British chemical workers exposed to formaldehyde. *J Natl Cancer Inst*, 95, 1608-1615.

Cogliano, V., Grosse, Y., Baan, R.A., Straif, K., Secretan, M.B. & El Ghissassi, F. (2005). Meeting report: summary of IARC monographs on formaldehyde, 2-butoxyethanol, and 1-tert-butoxy-2-propanol, *Environ. Health Perspect.* 113, 1205–1208.

Cole, P. & Axten, C. (2004). Formaldehyde and leukemia: an improbable causal relationship. *Regul. Toxicol. Pharmacol.* 40, 107–112.

COMEAP, Guidance on the Effects of Health of Indoor Air Pollutants, Committee on the Medical Effects of AirPollutants (2004). Available from: http://www.advisorybodies.doh.gov.uk/comeap/PDFS/guidanceindoorairqualitydec04.pdf.

Conaway, C., Whysner, J., Verna, L. & Williams, G. (1996). Formaldehyde mechanistic data and risk assessment: endogenous protection from DNA adduct formation. *Pharmacol. Ther.*, 71, 29 - 55.

Casanova, M., Heck, H.D., Everitt, J.I., Harrington, W.W.J. & Popp, J.A. (1988). Formaldehyde concentrations in the blood of rhesus monkeys after inhalation exposure. *Food Chem. Toxicol.* 26, 715–716.

Dreyfuss, J. (2010) Occupational formaldehyde exposure linked to increased risk of myeloid leukemia and death. *A Cancer Journal for Clinicians*, 60, 135-136.

Fenech, M., Holland, N., Chang, W., Zeiger, E. & Bonassi, S. (1999). The Human MicroNucleus Project - An international collaborative study on the use of micronucleus technique for measuring DNA damage in humans. *Mutat. Res.*, 428, 271 - 283.

Fenech, M., Chang, WP., Kirsch-Volders, M., Holland, N., Bonassi, S. & Zeiger, E. (2003). HUman MicronNucleus project: HUMN project: detailed description of the scoring criteria for the cytokinesis-block micronucleus assay using isolated human lymphocyte cultures. *Mutat Res*, 534, 65-75.

Goyer, N., Beaudry, C., Bégin, D., Bouchard, M., Buissonnet, S., Carrier, G., Gely, O., Gérin, M., Lavoué, J., Lefebvre, P., Noisel, N., Perrault, G. & Roberge, B. (2004). Impacts d'un abaissement de la valeur d'exposition admissible au formaldéhyde : industries de fabrication de formaldéhyde et de résines à base de formaldéhyde. Montréal : Institut de Recherche Robert-Sauvé en Santé et en Sécurité du Travail.

Granby, K., Christensen, CS. & Lohse, C. (1997). Urban and semi-rural observations of carboxylic acids and carbonyls. *Atmospheric Environment.* 31, 10, 1403-1415.

Hauptmann, M., Lubin, JH., Stewart, PA., Hayes, RB. & Blair, A. (2003). Mortality from lymphohematopoietic malignancies among workers in formaldehyde industries. *J. Natl. Cancer Inst.* 95, 1615–1623.

Hauptmann, M., Lubin, JH., Stewart, PA., Hayes, RB. & Blair, A. (2004). Mortality from solid cancers among workers in formaldehyde industries. *Am J Epidemiol.*, 159, 1117-1130.

Hauptmann, M., Stewart, PA., Lubin, JH., Beane Freeman, LE., Hornung, RW., Herrick, RF., Hoover, RN., Fraumeni, JF Jr., Blair, A. & Hayes, RB. (2009). Mortality from lymphohematopoietic malignancies and brain cancer among embalmers exposed to formaldehyde. *J Natl Cancer Inst.*, 101, 24, 1696-708.

He, J-L. & Jin, H.-Y. (1998). Detection of cytogenetic effects in peripheral lymphocytes of students exposed to formaldehyde with cytokinesis-blocked micronucleus assay. *Biomed. Environm. Sci.*, 11, 87-92.

Heck, H.D., Casanova-Schmitz, M., Dodd, P.B., Schachter, E.N., Witek, T.J. & Tosun, T. (1985). Formaldehyde (CH2O) concentrations in the blood of humans and Fischer-344 rats exposed to CH2O under controlled conditions. *Am. Ind. Hyg. Assoc. J.*, 46, 1–3.

Heck, H. & Casanova, M. (2004). The implausibility of leukemia induction by formaldehyde: a critical review of the biological evidence for distant-site toxicity. *Regul. Toxicol. Pharmacol.*, 40, 92–106.

Hildesheim, A., Dosemeci, M., Chan, CC., Chen, CJ., Cheng, YJ., Hsu, MM., Chen, IH., Mittl, BF., Sun, B., Levine, PH., Chen, JY., Brinton, LA. & Yang, CS. (2001). Occupational exposure to wood, formaldehyde, and solvents and risk of nasopharyngeal carcinoma. *Cancer Epidemiol Biomarkers Prev.*, 10, 1145-1153.

International Agency for Research on Cancer (IARC). (2006). *Formaldehyde, 2-Butoxyethanol and 1-tert-Butoxypropan-2-ol.* Lyon : IARC.

International Agency for Research on Cancer (IARC). (1985). *Tobacco Habits Other Than Smoking Betel-Quid and Areca-Nut Chewing and Some Related Nitrosamines.* Lyon : IARC.

International Programme on Chemical Safety (IPCS). (1991). Formaldehyde : health and safety guide. Geneva : World Health Organization. Available from: http://www.inchem.org/documents/hsg/hsg/hsg057.htm.

Kinney, P.L., Chillrud, S.N., Ramstrom, S., Ross, J. & Spengler, J.D. (2002). Exposures to multiple air toxics in New York City. *Environ. Health Perspect.*, 110 (Suppl. 4), 539–546.

Kromouht, H. (2002). Design of measurement strategies for workplace exposures. *Occup Environ Med.*, 59, 349-354.

Lubin, M., Stewart, JH., Hayes, PA. & Blair, RB. (2004). Mortality from solid cancers among workers in formaldehyde industries. *Am J Epidemiol.*, 159, 1117-1130.

Marsh, G.M. & Youk, A.O. (2004). Reevaluation of mortality risks from leukemia in the formaldehyde cohort study of the National Cancer Institute. *Regul. Toxicol.Pharmacol.* 40, 113–124.

Meijster, T., Tielemans, E., Schinkel, J. & Heederik, D. (2008). Evaluation of peak exposures in the Dutch flour processing industry: implications for intervention strategies. *Ann Occup Hy.*, 52, 587–596.

Mcglothlin JD. (2005). Occupational exposure assessment and control using video exposure monitoring in the pharmaceutical industry. Proceedings of International Scientific Conference (IOHA 2005), Pilanesberg National Park North West Province, South Africa. Pilanesberg September 2005.

Merk, O. & Speit, G. (1998). Significance of formaldehyde-induced DNA-protein crosslinks for mutagenesis. *Environ Mol Mutagen*, 32, 260-268.

NATIONAL INSTITUTE FOR OCCUPATIONAL SAFETY AND HEALTH (NIOSH) - NIOSH manual of analytical methods: DHHS (NIOSH) Publication 94-113. 4th ed. Atlanta, GA: Centers for Disease Control and Prevention, 1994.

Nazaroff, W., Coleman, BK., Destaillats, H., Hodgson, AT., Liu, D., Lunden, MM., Singer, BC. & Weschler, CJ. (2006). Indoor air chemistry: cleaning agents, ozone and toxic air contaminants. Berkeley, CA: Air Resources Board, California Environmental Protection Agency.

Nersesyan, A., Kundi, M., Atefie, K., Schulte-Hermann & R. Knasmüller, S. (2006). Effect of staining perocedures on the results of micronucleus assays with exfoliated oral mucosa cells. *Cancer Epidemiol Biomarkers Prev.*, 15, 1835 - 1840.

Odabasi, M. & Seyfioglu, R. (2005). Phase partitioning of atmospheric formaldehyde in a suburban atmosphere. *Atmospheric Environment.* 39, 28, 5149-5156.

Ohura, T., Amagai, T., Senga, Y. & Fusaya, M. (2006). Organic air pollutants inside and outside residences in Shimizu, Japan: levels, sources and risks. *Sci. Total Environ.* 366, 485–499.

Orsière, T., Sari-Minodier, I., Iarmarcovai, G. & Botta, A. (2006). Genotoxic risk assessment of pathology and anatomy laboratory workers exposed to formaldehyde by use of personal air sampling and analysis of DNA damage in peripheral lymphocytes. *Mutat Res.*, 605, 30-41.

Pinkerton, LE., Hein, MJ. & Stayner, LT. (2004). Mortality among a cohort of garment workers exposed to formaldehyde: an update. *Occup. Environ. Med.* 61, 193–200.

Preller, L., Burstyn, I., De Pater, N. & Kromhout, H. (2004). Characteristics of Peaks of Inhalation Exposure to Organic Solvents. *Ann Occup Hyg.*, 48, 643-652.

Pyatt, D., Natelson, E. & Golden, R. (2008). Is inhalation exposure to formaldehyde a biologically plausible cause of lymphohematopoietic malignancies? *Regulatory Toxicology and Pharmacology*, 51, 119–133.

Rosén, G., Andersson, IM., Walsh, PT., Clark, RD., Säämänen, A., Heinonen, K., Riipinen, H. & Pääkkönen, R. (2005). A review of video exposure monitoring as an occupational hygiene tool. *Annals of Occupational Hygiene.*, 1-17.

Ryan, TJ., Burroughs, GE., Taylor, K. & Kovein, RJ. (2003).Video exposure assessments demonstrate excessive laboratory formaldehyde exposures. *Applied Occupational and Environmental Hygiene.*, 18, 450-457.

SAC, Standardization Administration of China: Indoor Air Quality Standard. (2002). http://www.sac.gov.cn/templet/english/zmCountryBulletinByNoEnglish.do?countryBulletinNo=20021248.

Schwilk, E., Zhang, L., Smith, M., Smith, A. & Steinmaus, C. (2010) Formaldehyde and Leukemia: an updated meta-analyses and evaluation of bias. *Journal of Occupational and Environmental Medicine*, 52, 878-886.

Shaham, J., Bomstein, Y., Gurvich, R., Rashkovsky, M. & Kaufman, Z. (2003). DNA-protein crosslinks and p53 protein expression in relation to occupational exposure to formaldehyde. *Occup Environ Med.*, 60, 403-409.

Smith, T. (2001). Studying peak exposure: toxicology and exposure statistics. *In*: Marklund S., editor. X2001 - Exposure assessment in epidemiology and practice. Stockholm: National Institute for Working Life, 207-209.

Speit, G. & Schmid, O. (2006). Local genotoxic effects of formaldehyde in humans measured by the micronucleus test with exfoliated cells. *Mutat. Res.*, 613, 1-9.

Speit, G., Schmid, O., Fröhler-Keller, M., Lang, I. & Triebig, G. (2007). Assessment of local genotoxic effects of formaldehyde in humans measured by de micronucleus test with exfoliated buccal mucosa cell. *Mutation Research*, 627, 129-131.

Surrallés, J., Falck, G. & Norppa, H. (1996). In vivo cytogenetic damage revealed by FISH analysis of micronuclei in uncultured human T lymphocytes. *Cytogenet Cell Genet.*, 75, 151-154.

Suruda, A., Schulte, P., Boeniger, M., Hayes, RB., Livingston, GK., Steenland, K., Stewart, P., Herrick, R. ,Douthit, D. & Fingerhut, MA. (1993) Cytogenetic effects of formaldehyde exposure in students of mortuary science. *Cancer Epidemiol Biomarkers Prev.*, 2, 453-460.

Susi, P. & Schneider, S. (1995). Database needs for a task-based exposure assessment model for construction. *Applied Occupational Environmental Hygiene.*, 10, 394-399.

Tolbert, P., Shy, C. & Allen, J. (1991). Micronuclei and other nuclear abnormalities in buccal smears: a field test in snuff users, *Am. J. Epidemiol.*, 8, 840 - 850.

United States Environmental Protection Agency (USEPA). (2007). Indoor Air Quality (IAQ). Environmental Protection Agency. Available from: http://www.epa.gov/iaq/formalde.html.

Vaughan, TL., Stewart, PA., Teschke, K., Lynch, CF., Swanson, GM. & Lyon, JL. Berwick, M. (2000) Occupational exposure to formaldehyde and wood dust and nasopharyngeal carcinoma. *Occup Environ Med.*, 57, 376-384.

Viegas, S. & Prista, J. (2007). Cancro Nasofaríngeo e Exposição a Formaldeído: avaliação da história profissional em 63 casos registados. *Soc. Portuguesa de Medicina do Trabalho,* 6, 13-22.

Viegas, S. & Prista, J.(2010). Formaldehyde in Indoor Air: A Public Health Problem? *in Air Pollution XVIII.* 297-304. WIT Transactions on Biomedicine and Health. ISBN: 978-1-84564-450-5.

Vincent, R. & Jandel, B. (2006). Exposition professionnelle au formaldéhyde en France : informations fournies par la base de données Colchic. *Hygiène et sécurité du travail. Cahiers de notes documentaires.* 19-33.

WHO-ROE, Regional Office of Europe (2006). Development of WHO Guidelines for Indoor Air Quality World Health Organization. Available from: http://www.euro.-who.int/Document/AIQ/IAQ_mtgrep_Bonn_Oct06.pdf.

Wojda, A., Zietkiewicz, E. & Witt, M. (2007). Effects of age and gender on micronucleus and chromosome nondisjunction frequencies in centenarians and younger subjects. *Mutagenesis*, 22, 195-200.

Yao, X., Wang, W., et al. (2005). Seasonal change of formaldehyde concentration in the air of newly decorated houses in some cities of China. *J. Environ. Health,* 22, 353-355.

Ye, X., Yan, W., Zhao, M. & Ying, C. (2005). Cytogenetic analysis of nasal mucosa cells and lymphocytes from high-level long-term formaldehyde exposed workers and low-level short-term exposed waiters. *Mutation Research*, 588, 22-27.

Yokel, R. & MacPhail, R. (2011). Engineered nanomaterials: exposures, hazards, and risk prevention. *Journal of Occupational Medicine and Toxicology*. 21 -6:7.

Zhang, L., Steinmaus, C., Eastmond, D., Xianjun, K. & Martyn, T. (2009). Formaldehyde exposure and leukemia: A new meta-analysis and potential mechanisms. *Mutation Research*, 681, 150–168.

3

Ecological Risk Assessment on the Territory of Belarus After Chernobyl Accident

Irina Saltanova[1], Alexander Malenchenko[2] and Svetlana Sushko[2]
[1]*Joint Institute for Power and Nuclear Research "SOSNY",*
National Ac. Sci. of Belarus, Minsk,
[2]*Institute of Radiobiology,*
National Ac. Sci. of Belarus, Gomel,
Belarus

1. Introduction

Radiation contamination of several regions of Belarus was analyzed. As a part of analysis, statistical data on cancer cases was compared to the predicted data. Ecological situation due to chemical impact of industrial facilities' atmospheric releases was studied. For a biological model, an experimental study was carried out to investigate combined impact of radiation and chemical factors.

Complex assessment of radiation and chemical state was performed for 6 districts of Gomel region and 4 districts of Mohilev region. As the result of the assessment, model values for radiation and chemical risks were obtained.

In the relocation zone of Chernobyl Nuclear Power Plant (NPP), biological consequences of ecological factors (including radiation) combined impact were studied in a series of experiments. Laboratory mice of Af line (line of mice with high spontaneous frequency of lung tumors) were exposed in the relocation zone. The influence of exposure and natural background radiation level on the spontaneous and chemically induced process of lungs tumor development process was studied.

Linear risk assessment methodology proposed by the International Commission on Radiological Protection (ICRP) was used to analyze radiation risk. The US Environmental Protection Agency (EPA) methodology (with adjustments to local conditions) was used to analyze chemical risks.

2. Radiation risk assessment for Belarus regions which were most affected by Chernobyl accident

To assess health detriment of population of these regions, value of radiation induced injuries (probabilities of stochastic effects, which newly formed malignancies being the most dangerous) was used. Data on radiation risk assessment, as calculated according to linear non-threshold "Dose-effect" model, is presented in Table 1 for the Belarus territories most contaminated with radionuclide. In assessment, a lifelong risk coefficient for radiation induced cancers was used (5%/Sv, as suggested by *ICRP Recommendations*, 1990). The values of doses used for risk assessment were taken from *Compendium of Exposition Doses of Belarus Population* (1992). Therefore, the assessments presented determine possible cancers due to exposure at that period of time, and do not consider thyroid cancers induced by radiation and leukemia cases among the liquidators of the Chernobyl accident.

Location		**AEED*, mSv**	***R*, ×10⁻⁵**	***N***	n_p	Σn_p
Brahin	City	2.5	12.5	5635	0.704	2.1
	District	1.5	7.5	18083	1.356	
Vetka	City	3.1	15.5	9714	1.506	3.3
	District	2.1	10.5	16904	1.775	
Korma	City	2.0	10.0	6424	0.642	1.9
	District	1.7	8.5	15140	1.287	
Narovlya	City	2.3	11.5	11166	1.284	2.7
	District	3.4	17.0	8294	1.410	
Hoyniki	City	0.9	4.5	15813	0.712	2.5
	District	2.1	10.5	17015	1.787	
Chechersk	City	2.9	14.5	8915	1.293	2.8
	District	2.1	10.5	13986	1.469	

* - here, AEED is Annual Effective Equivalent Dose, *R* - risk, *N* - population, n_p - calculated values of found newly formed malignancies for a particular location, Σn_p - sum of n_p

Table 1. Radiattion risk assessment for Gomel region.

3. Carcinogenic risk analysis of environmental chemical contamination impact for Belarus regions which were most affected by Chernobyl accident

Quantitative connection between probability of sickness and dose of an individual is exposed is determined, when assessing risk from carcinogens. The value of risk may be presented in one of the following ways: as normalized risk per unit dose, as concentration risk corresponding to the given risk level, as individual risk, and as risk for a group of people. Knowing the values of individual risk allows predicting risk of cancer development at particular exposure values. Values of carcinogenic risks for the substances proven to be carcinogens at the locations in study are presented in Table 2. Calculated values of carcinogenic risk due to chemical contamination of the environment are presented in Tables 3 - 4 for two districts of Belarus.

Chemical compound	**Upper limit for risk**
Benzopyrene	7.3×10^{-12}
Bensol	7×10^{-6}
Formaldehyde	5×10^{-5}
Manganese	4×10^{-4}
Chromium	1.2×10^{-2}

Table 2. Additional lifelong cancer risk for a person weighting 70kg due to inhaling 1μg/m³ of a chemical compound during 70 years of life.

Region	Substance	C^*	R, ×10^{-5}	n per 10^5 people	N	n_p
Brahin	Manganese	0.32	1.82	1.8	23718	0.4
Vetka	Manganese	0.24	1.37	1.4	26618	0.4
Korma	Manganese	0.5	2.85	2.9	21564	0.6
Narovlya	Manganese Formaldehyde	0.05 0.36	0.29 0.08	0.3 0.1	19460	0.1
Hoyniki	Manganese Chromium	0.05 0.27	0.29 6.87	0.3 6.9	32828	2.4
Chechersk	Manganese	0.09	0.51	0.5	22901	0.1

* - concentration as fraction of Maximum Permissible Concentration (MPC)

Table 3. Calculated values of carcinogenic risk due to chemical contamination of the environment (Gomel district).

Predicted carcinogenic risk (both radiation and chemical) values were compares to eh statistical data on cancer sickness. In our work it is shown, that combined radiation and chemical contamination cannot be the source of detectable (above the background) carcinogenic risk. Impartial assessment of ecological risk can be developed only with the help of combined multifactor theoretical and experimental modeling.

Region	Substance	C^*	R	n per 10^5 people	N	n_p
Bykhov	Benzopyrene Bensol Chromium Formaldehyde	0.0015 0.003 0.3 0.2	1.56×10^{-13} 4.5×10^{-6} 7.71×10^{-5} 4.29×10^{-7}	≈0 0.45 7.71 0.043	53383	4.4
Krasnopol	Manganese Chromium	0.22 0.05	1.26×10^{-5} 1.29×10^{-5}	1.26 1.29	14720	0.4
Slavgorod	Benzopyrene Manganese Chromium	0.07 0.22 0.1	7.3×10^{-12} 1.26×10^{-5} 2.57×10^{-5}	≈0 1.26 2.57	19511	0.7
Chaussy	Benzopyrene Manganese	0.083 0.15	8.66×10^{-12} 8.57×10^{-6}	≈0 0.86	22716	0.2

* - concentration as fraction of Maximum Permissible Concentration (MPC)

Table 4. Calculated values of carcinogenic risk due to chemical contamination of the environment (Mogilev district).

It is obvious that the obtained estimates of additional sicknesses number (Tables 3 - 4) are maximal, as required by the general "ideology" of risk assessment.

4. Study of tumor formation in animals and their progeny when exposed to combined influence of ecological factors of different nature

Radiation effects may result not only from action of artificial radio nuclides, but from naturally occurring radioactive isotopes as well. Radioactive uranium isotopes, that are widely distributed, are accumulated in elevated amounts in organs of people, which live in goiter endemic regions of Belarus. Significant amount of enriched uranium from the wrecked unit of Chernobyl NPP got into the environment. So far, the issue of possible contribution of uranium and other naturally occurring radio nuclides to progeny inheritance of genetic system damages induced by radiation particularly or in the process of evolution have not been considered. However, this aspect of the issue has both a fundamental importance in analysis of natural radioactivity role and especial relevance for population of regions suffered from radiation damage, because total increased background radiation level has become a global ecological factor.

Discussed further, is a series of studies aimed on investigation of biological effects of joint influences of ecological factors.

Belarus population, which suffered from Chernobyl NPP accident and is now living on radiation-contaminated territory, form a group exposed to an increased risk of developing stochastic and genetic effects related to exposure (Spiridonov et al., 2007, Lorimore et al., 2005). One of the fundamental aspects of this problem is still to estimate stability of cells' genetic apparatus functioning, because damages to genome may become basis to immune system impairment, carcinogenesis, and decrease in life expectancy (Suskov et al., 2006).

Biological effects of joint influences of ecological factors, including radiation, can be most profoundly studied in the Chernobyl NPP relocation zone. Chernobyl NPP relocation zone is a unique place, where radiation is the dominating ecological factor, which is caused by the environment contamination level. The Polessky Radiation-Ecology Reserve (PRER) was created on this territory in 1988. Various radiobiological studies are carried out in PRER (Konoplya et al., 2011).

Series of studies were carried out in PRER to evaluate influence of:

1. Exposure on laboratory animals; and
2. Natural radioactivity on spontaneous and chemically induced tumor process in lungs (adenomas) of mice of Af line and their progeny (first generation - F1).

Usage of a biological model "lungs adenomas" as an accelerated test for Af-line mice to determine carcinogenicity of chemical substances is based on responsiveness in adenomas development under the action of various carcinogenic agents (Turusov and Parfenov, 1986). Mice used in the experiment are of "highly carcinogenic" Af-line, characterized by high sensitivity of lung tissue to blastomogenic effect of urethane and genetic predisposition to formation of tumors in lungs. Previously, urethane was widely used in pediatrics as a sedative measure. However, it was experimentally established that urethane causes a wide spectrum of embryonic disorders and tumors of different localization, independent of the way it was injected into body (Porubova, 2000).

Influence of exposure duration (1 and 4 months) in the Chernobyl NPP relocation zone on spontaneous and chemically induced mutagenesis and tumor formation in lungs of mice (Af line) and their progeny (first one - F1) was studied. The procedure of experiments was the following: male and female laboratory mice (3 month old) were delivered to the relocation zone in May 2007. Dose rate of 3.29 ± 0.10 µGy/hr was detected at the ground level where the mice were placed. After one month mice were split into the following groups: one part was relocated from the contaminated area to read background indicators, while the other part was allowed to copulate. Later pregnant females were relocated to vivarium in Minsk to get progeny F_1. In 24 hours after being relocated from the contaminated area, the animals were injected with urethane (1 mg/g, in the form of 10% sterilized solution with crystalline urethane - ethyl-carbonate, ($C_3H_7NO_2$) - Sigma - Aldrich). Animals were removed from the experiment after 72 hours after relocation from the contaminated area. 3-month old progeny F1 from parents, which were in the Chernobyl NPP relocation zone for 1 month, were injected with urethane (1 mg/g). Control was performed with the help of progeny F1 of the same age from Minsk vivarium. The same procedure was followed for laboratory animals after 4-month exposure in Chernobyl NPP relocation zone (PRER).

For parents and progeny, tumor process was assessed according to the number adenomas/mouse after 20 weeks of urethane injection. Influence of mice's uranium intoxication on sensitivity of the progeny to combined impact of exposure and urethane was studied by testing lungs adenomas. In this study, 3 weeks old immature male and female mice of Af line who were drinking solution of nitro-acid uranium ($UO_2(NO_3)_2{*}6\ H_2O$) in concentrations 180 mg/liter during the next 3.5 months, were used. (Novikov, 1974). After 3.5 months from the start of drinking, a part of animals, as well as control, were relocated for 7 - 10 days for copulation. Urethane (1 mg/g of body mass) was injected peritoneally to a part of immature animals 3.5 months after uranium intoxication as well as to intacted animals of the same age; adenomas were recorder after 20 weeks. Progeny of the intacted animals and 8- to 10-weeks old mice after uranium intoxication were exposed to 0.35 Gy gamma-rays (1 Gy/hr dose rate, ^{60}Co source), injected with urethane (1 mg/g), and exposed to combined radiation of the same dose and urethane concentration. Control was injected with the same amount of physiological solution. Tumor process was estimated by tumor rate (% of mice with adenomas) and adenomas/mouse number after 20 weeks according to the process described by Turusov and Parfenov (1986).

Experimental data were processed statistically using Student's criteria. An interaction coefficient K_w was used to describe quantitatively results of joint influence of factors of different origins. Interaction coefficient K_w was determined as a ratio of a system response to the combined radiation and toxic effect to the total effect of system responses to independent effects of individual factors (Kuzin, 1983). Effects were defined as and excess of level, induced by stressors, over spontaneous value. The result of interaction was considered to be additive if $K_w = 1$, and as antagonistic (synergetic) if K_w was reliably less (greater) than 1 (Geraskin et al., 1996).

The results of study of induced tumor process in lungs of mice (adenomas) placed in the relocation zone and in mice injected with urethane are presented in Table 5.

Analysis of results of influence of mice exposure in PRER zone on lung tumor process showed, that radio-ecological factors of Chernobyl NPP relocation zone increase tumors occurrence insignificantly (1.2 times) due to 1 months exposure, and increase tumors occurrence statistically significantly (more than 2.9 times) due to 4 months containment of animals in the zone. Also, intoxication of mice with urethane increases the number of adenomas in lungs statistically significantly for all the time period considered in the research.

Also, urethane injection to mice kept in Chernobyl NPP relocation zone for 1 and 4 months increases average adenomas/mouse number statistically significantly as compared to control. Interaction coefficient K_w was found to be 2.4 and 1.1 for mice exposed in the relocation zone during 1 and 4 months respectively. This signifies that joint effect of relocation zone factors and carcinogen (urethane) is synergetic, which decreases with exposure period in zone along with the increase in radiation contribution from 4.8 to 9.6%.

Exposure period	**1 month**			**4 months**		
Impact	**Mice number (male+ female)**	**Group-average number of adenomas / mouse**	K_w	**Mice number (male+ female)**	**Group-average number of adenomas / mouse**	K_w
Control (background level)	39	0.31 ± 0.09	–	27	0.26 ± 0.06	–
Urethane (Minsk vivarium)	26	7.03 ± 1.51*	–	27	3.36 ± 0.43*	–
Chernobyl NPP relocation zone	24	0.37 ± 0.02	–	22	0.77 ± 0.17*	–
Chernobyl NPP relocation zone + urethane	24	7.67 ± 2.08*8	2.4	21	8.05 ± 1.00*	1.1

* – Statistically significant difference from control-group, $p < 0.05$; ** – statistically significant difference from urethane control-group, $p < 0.05$.

Table 5. Number of induced adenomas/mouse in animals exposed in Chernobyl NPP relocation zone during 1 and 4 months.

Genome damages caused by the environment of Chernobyl NPP relocation zone are inherited by progeny. Originally, research of consequences of ionizing radiation influence for mammals was developing as studies of radiation effects for progeny of one exposed and one un-exposed parents. Thus, progeny was formed and developed from one exposed and one intact sex cell. However, since ionizing radiation became a global ecological factor, studies of radiation effects for progeny of parents who had been both exposed have become relevant. Studies of this problem have both fundamental and practical importance, because it has been neither unambiguously accepted, nor scientifically proven as to what dose to use to calculate genetic risk for progeny of both exposed parents (Nefedov et al., 2003).

Results of spontaneously and chemically induced carcinogenesis in lungs of F1 progeny of Af-line mice, both intact and exposed in PRER zone during 1 - 4 months, are presented in Table 6.

Evaluation of late effects showed that spontaneous occurrence of lungs adenomas had risen significantly (more than 5 times) for F1-mice progeny, that had been contained in Chernobyl NPP relocation zone during 1 month, as compared to the number of adenomas in lungs of progeny of intact mice.

Urethane injection to progeny of mice exposed in Chernobyl NPP relocation zone statistically significantly increases number of induced adenomas/mouse as compared to control-group (intact progeny of mice intoxicated with urethane).

Groups	Exposure period of mice-parents					
	1 months			4 months		
	Number of mice. n	Group average number of adenomas/mouse	K_w	Number of mice. n	Group average number of adenomas/mouse	K_w
F1 progeny (vivarium)	23	0.33 ± 0.07	-	34	0.23 ± 0.11	-
F1 progeny (vivarium + urethane)	25	6.10 ± 0.81*	-	26	6.38 ± 0.68*	-
F1 progeny of parents from Chernobyl NPP relocation zone	20	1.75 ± 0.61*	-	14	1.14 ± 0.36*	-
F1 progeny of parents from Chernobyl NPP relocation zone + urethane	14	10.28 ± 1.40*	1.38	14	8.85 ± 1.08*	1.22

* - Statistically significant difference from control-group, $p \leq 0.05$.

Table 6. Number of induced adenomas/mouse in F1 mice progeny that were exposed in Chernobyl NPP relocation zone during 1 and 4 months and/or were injected with urethane.

For F1-mice progeny which were exposed during 4 months in Chernobyl NPP relocation zone, the number of spontaneous tumors exceeded that for intact F1-mice progeny more than 4.9 times. Injection of urethane to F1-mice progeny, that had been previously exposed in Chernobyl NPP during 4 months, increased number of induced tumors by 7.76 times as compared to that of progeny of mice from Chernobyl NPP relocation zone (K_w = 1.22). It is important to notice an increased sensitivity of progeny of mice that had been exposed in Chernobyl NPP relocation zone, compared to their parents. This was pronounced in higher values of interaction coefficient K_w, namely, 1.38 – 1.22 with simultaneous decrease of radiation contribution from 17 to 12%.

A more pronounced difference in the level of induced tumor process occurred in the group of originally immature mice 6 months after stopping drinking uranium solution (adenomas/mouse number exceeded that of control-group more than 1.6 times). This signifies importance of age as a factor of animals' responsiveness to radiological and toxicological action.

Differences in responsiveness between intact animals and mice, which had been intoxicated with uranium, was also revealed while studying occurrences of tumors among animals after separate and joint uranium and urethane action, see Fig. 1.

Adenomas/mouse number increased statistically significantly after urethane action as compared to control-group ($p < 0.05$). Maximal value of tumor effect was observed among animals, which had been subjected to joint uranium and urethane action. This value exceeded level of urethane carcinogenesis more than by 10%, and reflects effect of combining influencing factors.

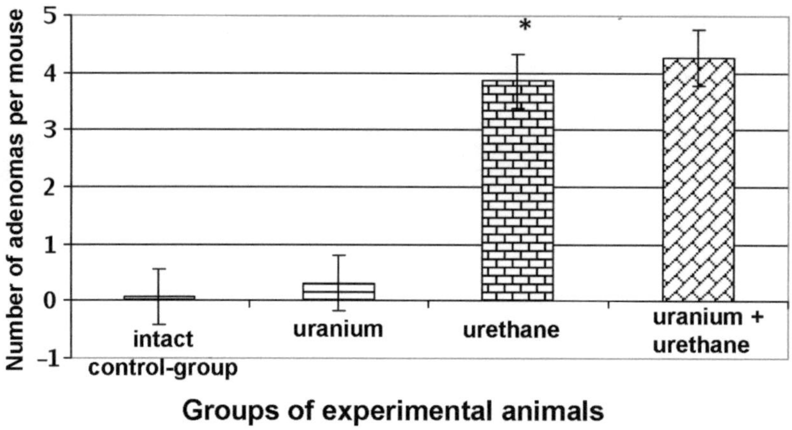

Fig. 1. Tumor formation among mice intoxicated with uranium (3.5 months) and being injected with urethane.

Apart from this, uranium intoxication as well as influence of low levels of various toxicants changes the responsiveness (sensitivity) of cells to the further action of different genotoxic factors. These changes manifest themselves in the form of a modifying effect, the exhibited level of the latter being determined by the level an organism is "familiar" with it.

Transgenetic transfer of sex cells; genome damages induced by uranium was also studied on Af-line mice. The results of studies are shown in Fig. 2.

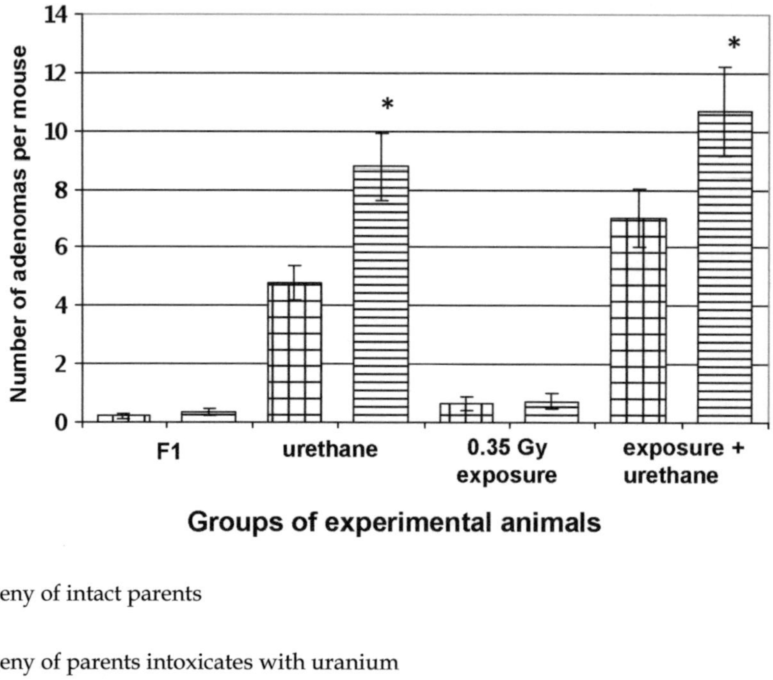

Fig. 2. Tumor formation and sensitivity of progeny (F1) of intact and intoxicated with uranium mice to exposure and chemical carcinogen.

Comparison of level in spontaneous tumor formations within progeny F1 of intact and intoxicated with uranium mice indicates a significant increase in adenomas/mouse number (more than by 63%) for progeny (F1) of mice that received nitric acid uranium (0.22 ± 0.09 and 0.36 ± 0.12 adenomas/mouse, respectively). Of a non-lesser importance is the difference in progeny sensitivity to the influence of additional agents. Urethane injection into progeny (F1) of uranium mice lead to statistically significant almost doubled (8.78 ± 1.17) increase in adenomas/mouse number that was observed within progeny of intact mice (4.77 ± 0.58). However, progeny responsiveness to exposure was somewhat different. In fact, the was almost no difference in number of induced adenomas/mouse between exposed progeny of uranium mice and that of exposed progeny of intact mice (0.72 and 0.66 adenomas/mouse) respectively. Subjecting to a joint effect of gamma-radiation and urethane group of progeny F1 of uranium mice, lead to the maximal (10.7 ± 1.52 adenomas/mouse) and statistically significantly exceeded the same indicator for a subjected to the joint effect of gamma-radiation and urethane group of progeny F1 of intact mice (7.05 ± 1.00 adenomas/mouse).

It follows from the obtained data, that:

1. Damages are induced in the genetic system of sex cells as a result of uranium intoxication;
2. These damages are transferred to progeny and manifest themselves as an increase in sensitivity of progeny to transformation under additional influence of genotoxic factors (i.e. genetic instability is induced).

Genetic instability may be one of the contributors to the formation mechanism of genetic burden.

4.1 Mathematical modeling of the consequences of the joint effect of the factors of radiation and non–radiation nature on the organism

Principles of the risk evaluation, used today for the population, residing on the territories, contaminated after the disaster at the Chernobyl NPP, are based mainly on the radiation influence analysis. However, results of the radiation risk assessment come into collision with the actually established changes in the quantity of the stochastic effects (officially published annual statistics), requiring an elaboration of new criteria of analysis that would be based on a multifactor influence.

In the framework of one of the problems of the present work, an attempt has been made to introduce a mathematical model of the synergic interaction of the factors of the radiation and non–radiation (on the example of a chemical carcinogen) nature and the damage manifestation as a result of such an interaction. A biological experiment has been carried out in the Radiation–Toxicological Ecology Laboratory of the Institute for Radio-Ecological Problems, National Academy of Sciences, Belarus (Malenchenko et al., 2001).

A hypothesis is proposed to create a mathematical model able to describe effects under a combined interaction, based on the assumption that a formation of additional effective damages takes place due to the interaction of subdamages, induced by each agent and not effective under a separate influence of each factors, both under combined and joint effect of any adverse environmental factors (Petin and Zhuravkovskaya, 1999).

Mathematical modeling of the consequences of the joint effect, based upon the above described method, turned out to be especially successful for a dose of 0.35 Gy owing to a monotonic character of the dependence "Number of the revealed damages" – "Time of the urethane introduction after the exposure to radiation". In accordance with the foregoing:

$$N_{\Sigma} = N_1 + PN_1, \quad (1)$$

where

N_{Σ} – total value of damages;

N_1 – amount of damages from the direct affect of the hazard factor (in our case – this is radiation);

P – share of "sub–damages", that are not revealed under a single radiation influence but reveal with addition of the second hazard factor (here – urethane).

Model (1) is stationary. If the sub–damages are not revealed under isolated influence of a single factor (radiation), then they will relax with time in the direction of the undamaged condition. We will consider this process as a purely probabilistic one with a constant relative rate (as in the case of the radioactive decay); i.e. the constant ratio of recoveries from the sub–damages rehabilitates per unit time. Then:

N_0 – amount of the damages from radiation;

PN_0 – amount of the sub–damages from radiation;

$PN_0 \cdot \exp(-t/\tau)$ – decreasing in the amount of sub–damages with time t and τ being "sub–damages lifetime".

Thus, we can find the amount of damages at any instant after irradiation under the urethane incorporation to be:

$$N(t) = N_0 + PN_0 \cdot \exp(-t/\tau), \quad (2)$$

where the second term of the sum is the amount of the sub–damages at the moment t, revealed as damages due to incorporation of the second hazardous factor (urethane).

On the basis of the experimental data, we are able to find average values of the parameters P and τ, corresponding to the experimental data with minimum error ε at the whole range of values:

$$P = 5.8 \pm 0.6 \ (\varepsilon \approx 10\%); \qquad \tau = 16 \pm 3 \text{ days } (\varepsilon \approx 20\%)$$

Hence, as for the dose of 0.35 Gy we get the following dependence of damages on time of the urethane incorporation after irradiation:

$$N(t) = 1.3 + 7.4 \cdot \exp(-t/16) \quad (3)$$

The modeled values shown in Fig. 3 were obtained in accordance with Eq. (3) and quite well correspond to the experimental values. This indicates a good fit of the model (2) to the experimental data in case of a monotonic character of dependence of the amount of damages on time.

Difficulty in getting an estimate for the tumor genesis process appraisal under combined action of radiation and chemical carcinogen is not only limited by the time period between interactions of carcinogens. Genesis of the radiation-induced tumor depends both on the dose and on its time distribution - the dose rate.

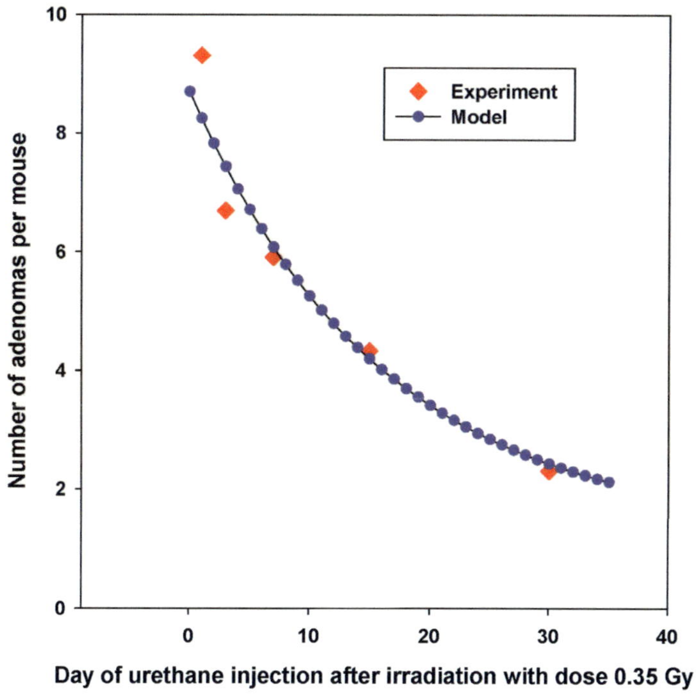

Fig. 3. Calculations according to model and experimental data.

Technical possibilities and latest experimental data allow revealing specific contribution of the radiation factor in the real ecological conditions and distinguishing single-factor risk due to radiation only. However, the attempt to extrapolate the findings for the current ecological conditions is connected with considerable difficulties that can mislead or show failure of the performed calculations. This was clearly pronounced in discrepancies between the predictions and the actual data on thyroid gland cancer occurrences among children in Belarus after the Chernobyl accident. In the view of this, we state that there is an obvious necessity to develop new methodological principles of the sanitary and ecological evaluation of the environmental quality under the conditions of joint effect of the ionizing radiation and factors of the non-radiation origin on human the organism.

5. Discussion

Currently, a special attention is paid to the issue of genome instability, which is caused by ionizing radiation. The main reason for this is that this issue is immediately related to understanding mechanisms of such important radiobiological phenomena as radiation mutagenesis, carcinogenesis, ageing, which are all remote consequences of ionizing radiation effects (Pelevina et al., 2003). Within concept of genome mutability, the phenomenon of genome instability induced by radiation is interpreted as a transition of progeny of exposed cells to the state of readiness to adaption changes. Such a state can have two outcomes: 1) adaptation to new conditions with a gradual normalization of cell systems and their functions by repairing and eliminating defective cells; or 2) transition to a modified state by means of preserved instability of genome; this can be accompanied by an occurrence of a malignant phenotype (Mazurik and Mikhaylov, 2001).

Obtained experimental data within out studies indicate that a combination of ecological factors present in Chernobyl NPP relocation zone induced damages in the sex cells genome of parents and promotes transgeneration transfer of these damages to the progeny. Obviously, similar process are occurring in organisms of animals and people that leave in contaminated areas that are close to Chernobyl NPP relocation zone. That's why, an increase of child sicknesses, that has been detected in recent years, may be not only a consequence of the current ecological situation, but also be a result of their parents being subjected to harmful to health effects after Chernobyl accident and accompanying adverse socio-economical and ecological factors (including naturally occurring radiation). These data pronounce an increase in the rate of genetic burden formation in organisms, subjected to the elevated radiation background level and influence of toxic factors. Such conditions are characteristic of territories suffered as the result of Chernobyl accident. Therefore, an impartial assessment of an ecological risk can be elaborates only be methods of combined multifactor theoretical and experimental modeling.

6. Conclusions

1. The radiation contamination due to Chernobyl accident cannot be the source of detectable carcinogenic risk on the territory of Belarus.
2. Current ideas about carcinogenic danger due to chemical contamination of the environment cannot be used for satisfactory explanation of the observed stochastic effects. Impartial assessment of ecological risk can be developed only with the help of combined multifactor theoretical and experimental modeling.
3. Combined-impact coefficient of interaction shows the mutually enhanced pattern of carcinogenic factors impact. The studied ecological factors induce damages to genome of parents' reproductive cells and its transgeneration transfer to the progeny.
4. Strategic aim of ecological risk studies is to solve the general problem: *to establish specific features and outputs of negative consequences (e.g. cancers) for human exposed to the specific combinations of technogenic and natural contamination.*

7. References

Compendium of Exposition Doses of Belarus Population (in Russian), 1992. Ministry of Health Care of Belarus, Research Institute for Radiational Medicine, 92 pages.

Heraskin, S.A., Dikarev, V.H., Udalov, A.A., et al., 1996. Influence of combined action of ionized radiation and heavy metals salts on occurrence of chromosome aberrations in spring barley's leaves meristem (in Russian), *Genetics*, vol. 32(2), pp. 279-288.

ICRP Recommendations, 1990. ICRP Publication 60, part 2, 1994 (Translated from English), Moscow, *Energoatomizdat* Publishing House, 207 pages.

Konoplya, Y.F., Vereshako, G.G., Goroh, G.A., Malenchenko, A.F., Sushko, S.N. et. al., 2011. *The effect of chronic radiation exposure of ChNNP Exclusion zone on the morfofunctional state and reactivity of organs and tissues of experimental animals,* chapter 14 in: *The lessons of Chernobyl: 25 years later,* Nova Science Publishers, pp. 1-13.

Kuzin, A.M., 1983. Transactions of Academy of Science of USSR (in Russian). *Biological series* 4, pp. 485 - 502.

Lorimore S.A., McIrath J.M., Coates P.J., et.al., 2005. Chromosomal instability in unirradiated hemopoietic cells resulting from a delayed in vivo bystander effect of gamma radiation, *Cancer Research,* vol. 65(13), pp. 5668-5673.

Malenchenko A.F., Sushko S.N., and Saltanova, I.V., 2003. Appraisal of irrational factors contribution depending on dose-effect and time-effect during the process of cancergenesis in combination of radiation ionization with chemical carcinogen, Proceedings of Fifth International Symposium and Exhibition on Environmental Contamination in Central and Eastern Europe, Institute for International Cooperative Environmental Research Florida State University. CD-ROM. - ISBN 0-9748192-0-4.- Prague, Czech Republic, 5 pages.

Malenchenko, A.F., Sushko, S.N., and Saltanova, I.V., 2001. Estimate of radiation factors contributionto "Dose-effect" and "Time-effect" dependences in the process of tumors formation during joint action of ionizing radiation and chemical carcinogen (in Russian), 2001. Annual "*Ecological anthropology*" published by *Belarusian committee "Children of Chernobyl"*, Minsk, Belarus, pp. 203-209.

Mazurik V.K., Mikhaylov, V.F., 2001. Radiation-induced genome instability: phenomenon, molecular mechanisms, and pathogenetic significance (in Russian), *Radiation biology. Radioecology,* vol. 41(3), pp. 272-289.

Nefedov, I.Yu., Nefedova, I.Yu., and Palyha, H.F.m 1996. Some methodological aspects of experimental modeling and estimation of consequences of exposing one and both parents (in Russian), *Radiation biology. Radioecology,* vol. 36(6), pp. 912-920.

Novikov, Yu.V., 1974. *Hygienic issues in studying uranium content in the environment and its influence on organism* (in Russian). Moscow, *Medicine* Publishing House, 231 pages.

Pelevina I.I., Aleshchenko, A.V., Antoshchina, M.M., et al., 2003. Response of a cells population to low-dose exposure (in Russian), *Radiation biology. Radioecology,* vol. 43(2), pp. 161-166.

Petin, V.H. and Zhuravkovskaya, H.P., 1999. *Synergy and environmental factors intensity* (in Russian), tutorial for students of specialty 013100 "Ecology", IPPE, Obninsk, Russia, 74 pages.

Porubova, H.M., 2000. Experimental study of genetic determination of a joint blastomogenic effect of a chronical low-dose ionizing radiation and a chemical carcinogen (in Russian), *Hygiene of populated areas,* vol. 2(36), Kiev, pp. 383-191.

Spiridonov, S.I., Aleksakhin, R.M., Fesenko, S.V., and Sanzharova, N.I., 2007. Chernobyl and the environment (in Russian), *Radiation biology. Radioecology,* vol. 47 (2), pp. 196-203.

Suskov, I.I., Kuzmina, N.S., Suskova, V.S., Baleva, L.S., and Sipyahina, A.E., 2006. Problem of induced genome instability as the basis of the increased sicknesses among child subjected to low-intensity influence of low-dose radiation (in Russian), *Radiation biology. Radioecology,* vol. 47(2), pp. 167-177.

Turusov, V.S., and Parfenov, Yu.D., 1986. *Methods of detection and regulation of chemical carcinogens* (in Russian), Moscow, 150 pages.

4

Focus on Bisphenol A, an Uncertain Environmental Pollutant

Salvatore Sciacca, Gea Oliveri Conti, Maria Fiore and Margherita Ferrante
University of Catania, Department "G.F. Ingrassia" Hygiene and Public Health, Italy

1. Introduction

Bisphenol A (BPA) is a ubiquitous chemical found in many consumer products. Despite the growing link between BPA and several diseases, including various cancers, it remains unregulated in many countries (like the USA).

BPA has a high industrial production-volume that started in the USA in 1957, but by 2001 was estimated to be globally approximately 2.5 million tons. It is widely used mainly in the production of polycarbonate (PC), plastics and epoxy resins, but also for many other applications (see Fig.1.) (Pfeiffer et al., 1997). Over 95% of BPA world consumption in 2009 was for those two purposes.

The PC applications include adhesives, compact disks, dental prosthesis and sealants, electrical and electronic parts, returnable empties, refillable water bottles and items for food such as sport bottles, baby bottles, pitchers, tumblers, home food containers and flatware. The epoxy applications include the protective coatings for the interiors and exteriors of food and beverage containers, as well as dental materials. BPA is also present in recycled and thermal paper (Keri et al., 2007; Ishido et al., 2004; Loffredo et al., 2010).

Because of those uses, consumers of canned food or infants being bottle fed are particularly exposed to BPA through their diet, though many other sources (environmental and occupational) of human exposure are proposed today by researchers.

BPA has drawn much discussion about its safety, due to its persistence in our environment (water, air, dust, waste sludge, food etc.) (Huang & Leung, 2009).

A variety of studies are available on BPA concentration in food (from food surveys) and BPA migration from contact with food including via baby bottles and dental materials, and BPA concentration in air, dust and water. There are also a limited number of studies available on BPA concentration in paper (FAO-WHO, 2010; Reuben, 2010).

A number of studies have involved BPA as a potential "endocrine disrupter," primarily on the basis of the results of in vitro exposure, that, however, have not been unequivocally confirmed in vivo.

Studies on the effects of BPA on health have focused on its oestrogenic activity, but some reports have also highlighted additional modes of its action, including liver damage, disrupted pancreatic β-cell function , thyroid hormone disruption and obesity-promoting effects (Karim & Husain, 2010; Keri et al., 2007).

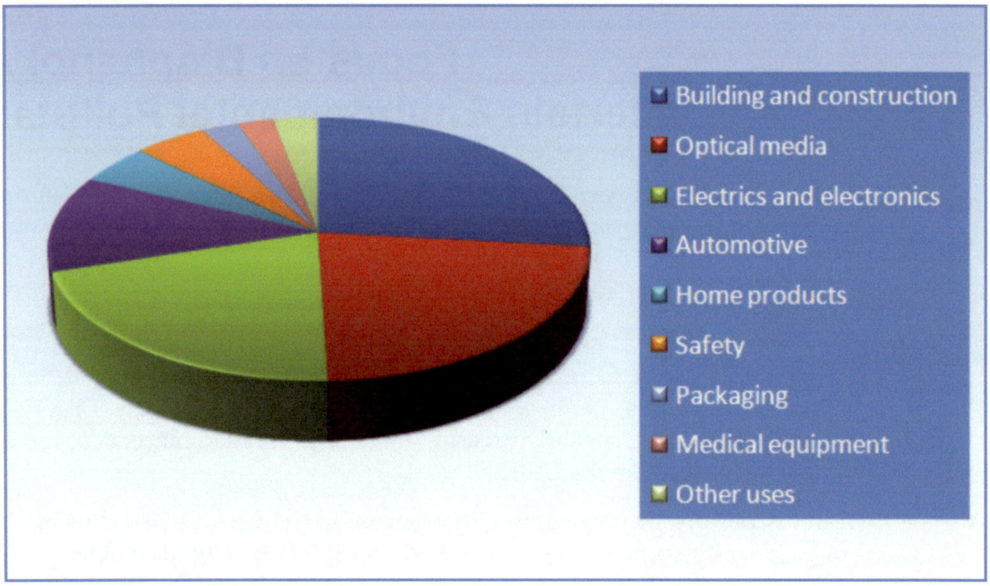

Fig. 1. European applications of BPA

BPA alters the cycle of the epithelial cells of the mammary gland in experimental mice and in human cells (in vitro) (Colerangle & Roy, 1997). It has received considerable media coverage, thus the problem is well known by the Western population, so much so that consumers have shown concern about BPA's oestrogenic effects.

All levels of government, from global to local, work to protect people from diseases through rigorous regulation of environmental pollutants (Dekant & Völkel, 2008; FAO-WHO, 2010). In the light of today's uncertainties about the possibility of the adverse human health effects at low doses of BPA exposure (especially on reproduction, the nervous system and behavioural development) and considering the relatively higher exposure of very young children compared with adults, the Food and Agriculture Organization of the United Nations (FAO) and the World Health Organization (WHO) jointly organised an expert meeting to assess the safety of BPA (FAO-WHO, 2010).

2. Bisphenol A

BPA, or 4,49-(1-methylethylethylidene) bisphenol, was first synthesised in 1905 (Fig. 2). It is obtained by condensation of phenol with acetone in the presence of a strongly acidic jelly-like ion-exchange resin as a catalyst.

Bisphenol A is a moderately water-soluble compound (300 mg/L at room temperature) and it dissociates in an alkaline environment (pK_a 9.9–11.3). It shows a weak acute toxicity for aquatic biota (Yamamoto et al., 2001).

It is used as a component of plastics, e.g. polyvinyl chloride, and as an antioxidant in glues, epoxy resins and ink.

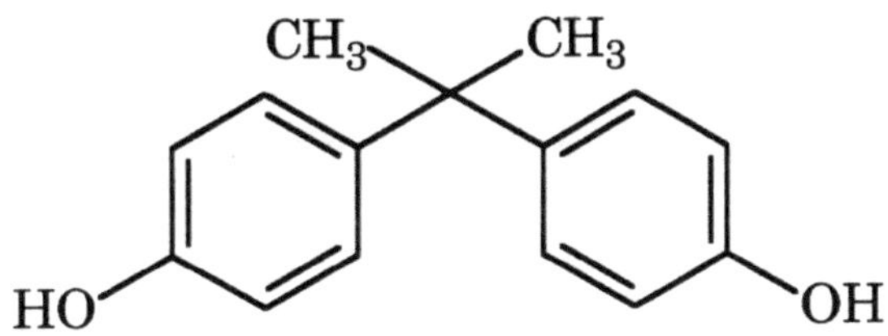

Fig. 2. Bisphenol A

Epoxy resins, in particular, are used as protective linings for a multitude of canned foods and beverages, and as a coating on metal lids for glass jars and bottles, including containers used for infant formula.

Materials containing BPA have been used for many applications in other packaging used for storage of food products, beverages and pharmaceuticals.

PC has been commonly used also for production of components of medical equipment (for dialysis and blood oxygenation), of returnable bottles for soft drinks, of infant feeding bottles, of kitchen dishes, toys, water pipes and polyethylene terephthalates or PET (Cobellis et al., 2009; Keri et al., 2007; Rykowska & Wasiak, 2006).

The wide use of polycarbonates arises mainly from their particular properties: light weight, durable, high tensile strength, very good elasticity, high melting point and high vitrification temperature (Rykowska & Wasiak, 2006).

2.1 Exposure routes to BPA

It is important to note that the border line between occupational and environmental contaminants is very fine and often difficult to demarcate with accuracy.

Many known or suspected carcinogens, in fact, were first identified by studying industrial and agricultural occupational exposures, while later they were found in the environment and in numerous consumer products.

Human exposure to BPA may arise, then, also out of BPA leaching from those materials into the saliva or may occur through skin contact (Cobellis et al., 2009; Keri et al., 2007; Takahashi et al., 2001).

Generally, higher doses are found in small groups due to exposure in their workplace, whereas environmental exposures are found at lower doses but in large populations.

Very few studies have been done on the environmental occurrence of BPA. Recently, the Environment Agency of Japan reported that environmental pollution by BPA is widespread in Japan. BPA has been, in fact, also found in sediments and fish (Yamamoto et al., 2001).

Many studies show that levels detected in beverages are lower than levels in food, levels in fruits are lower than in vegetables, while levels in fatty foods are higher than levels in all other foods. Data also exist on BPA levels in tap water and bottled water (FAO-WHO, 2010).

BPA concentrations in air and dust are widely distributed and there is no difference between indoor and outdoor air.

Few studies have been carried out on BPA in paper packaging, paper treatment water and thermal paper. BPA levels were detected higher in recycled paper than in virgin paper, therefore, additional studies on BPA migration from paper packaging to food are needed (FAO-WHO, 2010).

When waste plastics containing BPA are buried in a landfill a hydrolytic or leaching process may occur to release the BPA from waste to leachate. Landfill leachates are therefore also an important source of environmental BPA (Yamamoto et al., 2001).

As BPA can arise out of those sources, human exposure to this compound occurs especially in urbanised and industrialised areas.

EFSA in 2006 set the Tolerable Daily Intake (TDI) at 0.05 mg BPA/kg body weight (b.w.)/day.

In 2008, EFSA, following more recent studies, reaffirmed the same TDI (EFSA, 2010).

Small amounts of BPA can potentially leach out from food containers into foodstuffs and beverages, and therefore be ingested; as a consequence, in the European Union (EU), BPA is permitted in plastics for food only if the specific migration limit of 0.6 mg/kg of food is respected (see Directive 2002/72/EC relating to plastic materials and plastic materials intended to come into contact with food).

The use of BPA in food contact materials is also authorised in other countries like the USA and Japan.

The new EU implementing Regulation No 321/2011, has replaced Directive 2002/72/EC, making it clear that BPA is "not to be used for the manufacture of polycarbonate baby bottles for feeding infants".

Although FDA and EFSA ruled in 2008 that BPA is safe even for infants, in the same year Canada took a precautionary approach classifying BPA as ''toxic'' under the Canadian Environment Protection Act and it has banned its use in baby bottles and infant formula cans. More than 20 states in the USA are following suit with proposed or enacted BPA bans.

In January 2010, FAO acknowledged that there is concern about BPA's effects, but concluded that there was insufficient scientific evidence to support a product ban or even a requirement to label BPA-containing products.

Endocrine disruptors (EDs) represent a major toxicological and public health issue.

Endocrine disruptors are an extensive group of natural or anthropogenic organic molecules that act as hormone-like substances; they are widely dispersed in the environment and are capable of mimicking the action of steroidal oestrogens (Keri et al., 2007; Ishido et al., 2004; Loffredo et al., 2010).

Among endocrine disruptors BPA is a known xenoestrogen (Ishido et al., 2004).

Studies in vivo have shown that BPA can mimic 17β-estradiol in stimulating prolactin secretion, inducing growth and differentiation and exhibiting uterotrophic activity in rats and mice (Ishido et al., 2004), however, BPA oestrogenicity in vitro has been observed to be 15,000 times less active than 17β-estradiol.

It is important to highlight that oestrogens are important in the maintenance of human pregnancy and the placenta is its major site. BPA is capable of potentially reducing oestrogen synthesis by down-regulating CYP of placental cells (Huang & Leung ,2009).

Studies of prenatal exposure to BPA have shown in mice changes of the gross ovarian anatomy (a reduction in the number of corpora lutea and an increase in unilateral or bilateral ovarian bursae). Others have reported that BPA exposure increases aneuploidy and this has been linked to miscarriages also in humans (Huang & Leung, 2009).

2.1.1 Environmental exposures to BPA

Assessing health hazards due to drinking water contamination is difficult, since it is usually challenging to estimate the levels and timing of exposures, and the specific chemicals involved. It can also be difficult to clearly define exposed populations. Furthermore, it is often not possible to identify the cause of observed health effects when there are multiple exposures or to link specific health effects with an individual chemical that occurs in mixtures (FAO-WHO, 2010; Reuben 2010; Sciacca & Oliveri Conti, 2009).

Many bottled water users assume that it is cleaner than tap water, but BPA can leach from the bottle itself into the water it contains (Reuben, 2010).

Due to the low BPA vapour pressure, inhalation exposure of the general population will likely have only a minor contribution compared to the overall exposure. Inhalation of household dust containing BPA is unlikely to result in significant uptake of BPA from the lung because the large particles typically encountered in household dust do not penetrate into the low lung. However, house dust may be trapped in the mucociliary layer and may be swallowed resulting in additional oral exposure.

Indirect ingestion (dust, soil and toys) is considered to be approximately 0.03 µg/kg bw per day in infants and approximately 0.0001 µg/kg bw per day in children and adults (FAO-WHO, 2010).

Non-occupational dermal exposures to BPA are considered as rare events, moreover, systemic bioavailability of BPA after dermal application is limited to only 10%.

The mean exposure from inhalation of free BPA (concentrations in indoor and outdoor air) is approximately 0.003 µg/kg bw per day for the general population (FAO-WHO, 2010).

Based on this evidence, several government organisations have concluded that oral exposure through food is the major source for BPA exposure in all age groups of non-occupationally exposed human subjects (Reuben, 2010).

Some additional oral exposure to BPA may also result from using BPA-based resins in dentistry, but this is restricted to a short period after treatment with BPA-based dental sealants or composites.

Due to the wide range of applications of BPA in food cans and materials for packaging for food commodities, food may significantly contribute to human BPA exposure.

The EU estimated daily exposures to BPA from a minimum of 0.02 µg/kg bw/day to 59 µg/kg bw/day in adults. The EFSA estimated intakes of BPA through food from 0.2 µg/kg bw/day (a three month old infant fed with only breast milk) to 13 µg/kg bw/day (a six month old infant fed with polycarbonate bottles and commercial food). Exposures to BPA based on direct food analysis and food consumption patterns generally resulted in estimates of low daily human exposure ranging from 0.005 to 0.37 µg/kg bw/day (Dekant & Völkel, 2008; EFSA, 2010; FAO-WHO, 2010; Reuben, 2010).

2.1.2 Foetal exposure to BPA

Recent data from epidemiological studies have suggested that perturbations in the foetal environment may predispose individuals to disease and/or organ dysfunction, that becomes apparent in adulthood.

This theory on the foetal origins of adult diseases has prompted scientists to hypothesise that foetal exposure to environmental oestrogens has increased incidence of uterine leiomyoma, testicular cancer and breast cancer as observed in European and US populations over the last 50 years.

Exposure of rodents to low doses of BPA during foetal development has been shown to alter a variety of biological endpoints including early vaginal opening, early onset of puberty, disrupted oestrous cyclicity and decreased levels of luteinising hormone after ovariectomy. These results give strong credence to the supposition that there is a link between foetal exposure to BPA and the development of neoplasias in the adult mammary gland.

These neoplasias may have their origin in the altered morphogenesis that occurs in the foetus during the period of BPA exposure (FAO-WHO, 2010; Murray et al., 2007; Reuben, 2010).

Emerging evidence is that BPA affects the developing brain in the foetus, leading to severe behavioural alterations. Therefore, the hypothesis that BPA might also contribute to the incidence of neurodevelopmental disorders such as attention deficit, hyperactivity disorder and autism has been posited (Ishido et al., 2004).

However, for EFSA, the foetal exposure and also the exposure to total BPA through lactation appear to be limited (EFSA, 2010).

The recent final report of the US National Toxicology Program (NTP) stated that "*there is currently insufficient evidence to conclude that Bisphenol A exposure during development predisposes laboratory animals to develop obesity or metabolic diseases such as diabetes, later in life...*" (EFSA, 2010; Reuben; 2010).

2.1.3 Potential dietary exposure for infants aged 0 to 3

The estimated maximum BPA migration from PC baby bottles is 15 µg/kg. This intake is considered to be safe for consumers.

Infants fed with canned liquid formula in PC bottles, were exposed to 4.5 µg/kg bw per day with a mean of 2.4 µg/kg bw per day, whereas infants fed with powdered formula (prepared when needed) were exposed to lower levels (2.7 µg/kg bw per day with a mean of 2.0 µg/kg bw).

When infants were fed with canned liquid formula in PC-free bottles, the estimates were 0.5 µg/kg bw per day at the mean and 1.9 µg/kg bw per day at the 95th percentile, whereas the estimates were lower, 0.01 and 0.1 μg/kg bw per day, respectively, for infants fed with powdered formula.

Therefore, the difference between canned liquid and powdered formula is mainly caused by the migration of BPA from the epoxy resin coating the cans in which liquid formula is packaged.

Hence, it has been estimated that the major sources of exposure in this age group are:

- migration of BPA from PC bottles (81%),
- infant liquid formula packaged in PC containers or metal cans with epoxy linings (19%),
- epoxy resin in contact with powdered milk formula (1%).

For children aged 3 and older, the main source of exposure is instead migration from canned food that contributes to 94% of the total exposure (FAO-WHO, 2010).

3. Metabolism and toxicokinetics

BPA is well absorbed from the gastrointestinal tract with conversion to Bispenol A - glucuronides and Bispenol A-sulphate; this phase is critical but not very important because unlike the aglycone-BPA (i.e. free or unconjugated) BPA- glucuronides does not bind to the oestrogen receptor (see Fig.3). Aglycone-BPA does not accumulate in the body.

Glucuronide-BPA is subjected to biliary excretion, enterohepatic recirculation and principally to faecal excretion; humans excrete conjugated forms of BPA in the urine within 6 h (see Fig.3) (FAO-WHO, 2010; Keri et al., 2007).

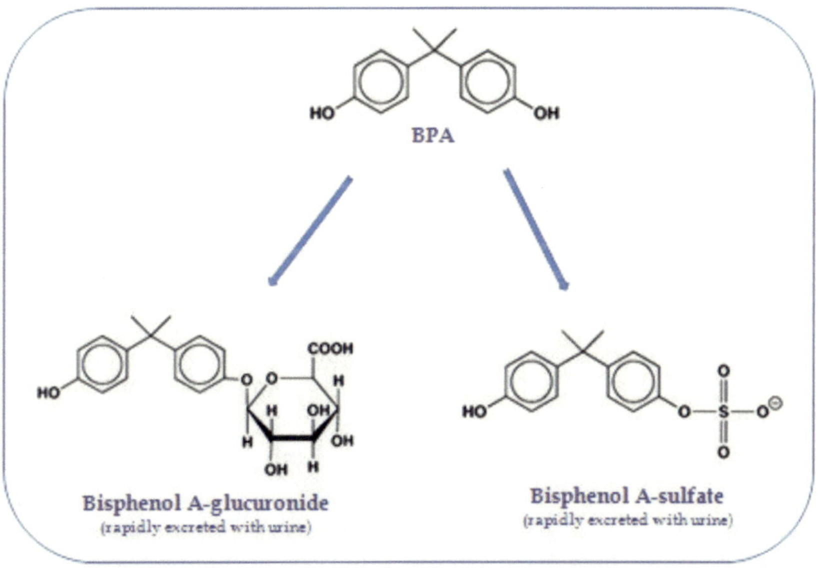

Fig. 3. Biotransformation of bisphenol A in humans to bisphenol A-glucuronide and bisphenol A-sulfate.

4. Mutagenicity and genotoxicity of BPA

Nitrosylation reactions have been associated with the production of several carcinogens, many of which elicit cancers in humans and animals.

Several mutagens have been found by nitrosation of phenol derivatives present in several foodstuffs, including soy sauce, smoked foods, etc.

It has been proven that BPA can be activated into a mutagenic species through nitrosylation reactions, raising the possibility that migration of BPA from polycarbonate or epoxy-lined containers into nitrite-containing foodstuffs could lead to the formation of mutagenic compounds. There is also the possibility that ingestion of BPA in addition to a nitrite-rich diet could lead to the production of mutagens. However, this contribution of nitrosylated-BPA is a new hypothesis of carcinogenesis that is still speculative.

No epidemiological studies have found that BPA is correlated with cancer incidence in the human population, especially with gastric or oesophageal cancers that can be indicative of dietary exposure to nitrosylated mutagens.

The native BPA is non-mutagenic, however the incubation of BPA with sodium nitrite in an acidic environment activates the BPA into a direct-acting frameshift type and base pair mutagen in a variety of sites of nucleic acid in the Ames Salmonella assay (Schrader et al., 2002).

It has been stated that BPA is not likely to pose a genotoxic hazard to humans (FAO-WHO 2010; Keri et al., 2007), although there is only limited data available on the genotoxicity of BPA in human cells (Takahashi et al., 2001).

5. Carcinogenicity of BPA

There are no human epidemiology studies in the existing literature that have produced relevant data for the assessment of the carcinogenic potential of BPA (Haighton et al., 2002). BPA may be associated with increased cancers of the haematopoietic system, breast and a significant increase in interstitial-cell tumours of the testes. DNA adducts generally are formed in target mammary cells. Although DNA adducts do not necessarily evolve into tumours or other chronic degenerative diseases, the formation of these molecular lesions in target mammary cells may have relevance for the potential involvement of BPA in breast carcinogenesis (Izzotti et al., 2009). In addition to forming DNA adducts itself, BPA may act indirectly by unbalancing oestrogen metabolism; these effects could be additive, increasing even further the risk of BPA to initiate cancer (Cavalieri & Rogan, 2010).

BPA alters microtubule function and can induce aneuploidy in some cells and tissues. It has been speculated that the ability of BPA to induce aneuploidy may play a role in the development of cancer (Takahashi et al., 2001) but also low doses of BPA generate reactive oxygen species (ROS) by decreasing the activities of antioxidant enzymes and increasing lipid peroxidation, thereby causing oxidative stress in the liver of rats (Bindhumol et al., 2003).

Extensive research has revealed that the oxidative stress can lead to chronic inflammation, which in turn could mediate most chronic diseases including cancer, diabetes and cardiovascular, neurological and pulmonary diseases. The oxidative stress activates the inflammatory pathways leading to transformation of a normal cell to tumour cell (Kamp et al., 2011; Reuter et al., 2010).

Early life exposure to BPA may induce or predispose to preneoplastic lesions of the mammary gland and prostate gland in adult mice, but this is not yet demonstrated in humans; also prenatal exposure to environmental doses of BPA alters the mammary gland development in mice, increasing the endpoints considered markers of breast cancer risk in humans. Investigators funded by the US National Institutes of Health (NIH) concluded that a strong correlation is found between the above-named exposure, cancer and early puberty. Several studies aimed at demonstrating the increases of some tumour types after BPA exposure were considered not to provide convincing evidence for carcinogenicity.

BPA exposure during the perinatal period is important because it has been hypothesised that it could alter the prostate and mammary gland development, predisposing to neoplastic or preneoplastic conditions (see section 2.1.2) (EFSA; 2010; FAO-WHO, 2010).

In any case the European Commission, in addition to known carcinogens, includes BPA in the lists of chemicals that are "of concern".

6. Reproductive and developmental toxicity of BPA in mammalian species

Emerging evidence has proposed a putative role for ubiquitous environmental contaminants in the occurrence of endometriosis. The mechanism of action may be carried out through the interaction with steroidal receptors, mimicking an oestrogenic effect (Cobellis et al., 2009).

Bisphenol A has been proven to have oestrogenic activity, even at concentrations below 1 ng/L. A study on mice revealed that a concentration of BPA as low as 20 ppm in drinking water is sufficient to bring about genetic changes in mice foetuses. The changes are a result of disturbance of the distribution of chromosomes in the daughter cells (Rykowska & Wasiak, 2006). The US Center for the Evaluation of Risks to Human Reproduction concluded in 2008 that there is "some concern for effects on the brain, behaviour, and prostate gland in foetuses, infants, and children at current human exposures to bisphenol A".

Several governing agencies, recently, have identified an oral reproductive and developmental NOAEL of 50 mg/kg bw per day (FAO-WHO, 2010).

7. Conclusions

Much remains to be learned about the effects of BPA environmental exposure on cancer risk. Based on what is known, however, there is much that governments and industry can do now to address or prevent environmental cancer risk.

At the same time, individuals can take important steps in choices of lifestyle to reduce their exposure to environmental elements that increase risk of cancer and other severe diseases.

Furthermore, the individual's small actions, if considered collectively, can drastically reduce the number and levels of environmental contaminants.

Some alternatives to BPA-containing materials for PC bottles and containers, and epoxy can linings are available on the world's market or proposed for domestic use. The functionality and safety of any replacement material need to be carefully assessed before use or sale.

However, as it appears that it will not be possible to identify a single replacement for all uses of BPA, particularly for can coatings, the problem is still open.

Due to the gaps in the current literature, it is premature to conclude that BPA is certainly a carcinogenic, however, the evidence suggests that BPA increases cancer susceptibility through developmental reprogramming and changes in target organ morphogenesis as a result of epigenetic alterations. It is important to underscore that studies examining changes in carcinogenic susceptibility have only focused on the mammary and prostate glands, two obvious targets of potential endocrine disruption, but it is necessary to include vagina, uterus, ovary and testes.

Usually, the main exposure route for humans to low environmental doses of BPA is orally. There is no doubt that BPA is an environmental pollutant, although it is not yet considered a carcinogen, therefore the ALARA (As Low As Reasonably Achievable) concept should be employed for protection of consumers and the general population.

8. Acknowledgments

The authors gratefully acknowledge the contribution of Dr. Pasquale Di Mattia in terms of comments, medical English and constructive suggestions provided for improving the manuscript.

9. References

Bindhumol, V., Chitra, K.C., Mathur, P.P. (2003). Bisphenol A induces reactive oxygen species generation in the liver of male rats. *Toxicology*; 188:117-124.

Cavalieri, E.L., Rogan, E.G. (2010). Hypothesis. Is Bisphenol A a Weak Carcinogen like the Natural Estrogens and Diethylstilbestrol? *Life*; 62(10): 746–751.

Cobellis, L., Colacurci, N., Trabucco, E., Carpentiero, C., Grumetto, L. (2009). Measurement of bisphenol A and bisphenol B levels in human blood sera from healthy and endometriotic women. *Biomed. Chromatogr.*; 23: 1186–1190.

Colerangle, J.B., Roy, D., (1997). Profound effects of the weak environmental Estrogen-like chemical Bisphenol A on the Growth of the mammary gland of Noble rats. *J. Steroid Biochem. Molec. Biol.*; Vol. 60, N°. 1-2, pp 153-160.

Dekant, W., Völkel, W. (2008). Human exposure to bisphenol A by biomonitoring: methods, results and assessment of environmental exposures. *Toxicology and Applied Pharmacology;* 228 : 114–134.

European Food Safety Authority (EFSA) (2010). Scientific Opinion on Bisphenol A: evaluation of a study investigating its neurodevelopmental toxicity, review of recent scientific literature on its toxicity and advice on the Danish risk assessment of Bisphenol A1. *EFSA Journal*; 8(9):1829.

FAO-WHO (2009). *Bisphenol A (BPA) - Current state of knowledge and future actions by WHO and FAO. INFOSAN Information Note* No. 5/2009 - Bisphenol A.

FAO-WHO (2010). *Joint FAO/WHO Expert Meeting to Review Toxicological and Health Aspects of Bisphenol A*. 1-5, November 2010, Ottawa, Canada.

Kamp, D.V., Shacter, E., Weitzman, S.A. (2011). Chronic inflammation and cancer: the role of the mitochondria. *Oncology*; 25(5): 400-10,413.

Karim, Z., Husain Q. (2010). Application of fly ash adsorbed peroxidase for the removal of bisphenol A in batch process and continuous reactor: assessment of genotoxicity of its product. *Food and Chemical Toxicology*; 48: 3385–3390.

Keri, R.A., Ho, S.M., Hunt, P.A., Knudsen, K.E., Soto, A.M., Prins, G.S. (2007). An Evaluation of Evidence for the Carcinogenic Activity of Bisphenol A. *Reprod Toxicol.*; 24 (2): 240–252.

Haighton, L.A., Hlywka, J.J., Doull, J., Robert, K., Lynch, B.S., Munro, I.C. (2002). An Evaluation of the Possible Carcinogenicity of Bisphenol A to Humans. *Regulatory Toxicology and Pharmacology*, 35: 238–254.

Huang, H., Leung, L.K. (2009). Bisphenol A downregulates CYP19 transcription in JEG-3 cells. *Toxicology Letters*, 189:248–252.

Ishido, M., Masuo, Y., Kunimoto, M., Oka, S., Morita, M. (2004). Bisphenol A causes hyperactivity in the rat concomitantly with impairment of tyrosine hydroxylase immunoreactivity. *Journal of Neuroscience Research*; 76:423–433.

Izzotti, A., Kanitz, S., D'Agostini, F., Camoirano, A., De Flora, S.(2009). Formation of adducts by bisphenol A, an endocrine disruptor, in DNA in vitro and in liver and mammary tissue of mice. *Mutation Research/Genetic Toxicology and Environmental Mutagenesis*; Vol 679, Issue 1-2, pp 28-32.

Loffredo, E., Gattullo, C.E., Traversa, A., Senesi, N. (2010). Potential of various herbaceous species to remove the endocrine disruptor bisphenol A from aqueous media. Chemosphere 80:1274–1280.Murray, T.J., Maffini, M.V., Ucci, A.A., Sonnenschein, C., Soto, A.M. (2007). Induction of mammary gland ductal hyperplasias and carcinoma in situ following fetal bisphenol A exposure. *Reproductive Toxicology*; 23: 383–390.

Pfeiffer, E., Rosenberg, B., Deuschel, S., Metzler, M. (1997). Interference with microtubules and induction of micronuclei in vitro by various bisphenols. *Mutation Research*; 390 : 21–3.1

Reuben, S.H., (2010). Reducing Environmental Cancer Risk. What We Can Do Now. *2008–2009 Annual Report*. President's Cancer Panel. US Department of Health and Human Service. National Institutes of Health. National Cancer Institute.

Reuter, S., Gupta, S.C., Chaturvedi, M.M., Aggarwal, B.B. (2010). Oxidative stress, inflammation, and cancer: how are they linked? *Free Radic. Biol. Med.*;49(11):1603-16.

Rykowska, I., Wasiak, W. (2006). Properties, Threats, and methods of analysis of Bisphenol A and its derivatives. *Acta Chromatographica*, No. 16, pp 7-27.

Schrader, T.J., Soper, K., Langlois, I., Cherry, W. (2002). Mutagenicity of Bisphenol A (4,4'-Isopropylidenediphenol) In Vitro: Effects of Nitrosylation. *Teratogenesis, Carcinogenesis, and Mutagenesis*; 22: 425–441.

Sciacca, S., Oliveri Conti, G. (2009). Mutagens and carcinogens in drinking water. *Mediterranean Journal of Nutrition and Metabolism*; 2:157-162.

Takahashi, S., Chi , X.J., Yamaguchi , Y., Suzuki, H., Sugaya, S., Kita, K., Hiroshima, K., Yamamori, H., Ichinose, M., Suzuki, N. (2001). Mutagenicity of bisphenol A and its suppression by interferon-α in human RSa cells. *Mutation Research*; 490: 199–207.

Yamamoto, T., Yasuhara,A., Shiraishi,H., Nakasugi O. (2001). *Bisphenol* A in hazardous waste landfill leachates. *Chemosphere;* 42:415-418.

Section 3

Test for Detection of Carcinogens

5

The Ty1 Retrotransposition Short-Term Test for Selective Detection of Carcinogenic Genotoxins

Teodora Stoycheva[1], Margarita Pesheva[2],
Martin Dimitrov[2] and Pencho Venkov[1]
*[1]Institute of Cryobiology and Food Technology,
Department of Cryobiology and Lyophilization, Sofia,
[2]Sofia University, Faculty of Biology, Department of Genetics, Sofia,
Bulgaria*

1. Introduction

A number of breakdowns in human's health including cancer have been attributed to the exposure of environmental pollutants, and it became imperative to check the potential toxicity, mutagenicity or carcinogenicity of a number of chemicals. The tests designed for such studies are divided into long-term and short-term assays.

Long-term tests are bioassays for carcinogenicity using animals (mainly rats or mice) as testers. Targets of the carcinogenic action are either organs or the whole body of the tester animal studied by dissection and histochemical analysis. These bioassays are not suitable for the study of a large number of substances because they are time consuming, expensive, require special facilities and qualified personal. A full long-term assay is completed in an average period of two years which stimulated the development of medium-term bioassays (Ito et al. 1998). These assays determine formation of neoplasms in various tissues of rats or mice within a period of 12-18 months. However, the existence of thousands genotoxins with potential carcinogenic effect requires the application of much faster assays and short-term tests have been developed and widely used. According to the timeframe required to obtain results in an assay, the transgenic mouse systems are intermediate between long-term and short-term tests. Although designated as "short-term bioassays" (Tennant et al. 1995) results from these tests are obtained in 4-6 months. The modified genes of transgenic animals cause them to respond rapidly to carcinogens (Cannon et al. 1997). Transgenic mouse systems are statistically reliable *in vivo* assays and the positive results obtained in the tests are highly predictive of rodent carcinogenicity.

1.1 Advantages of short-term tests

Short-term tests identify genotoxic agents by detecting the three major end-points associated with human cancer diseases: gene mutation, clastogenicity and aneuploidy. The main value of the short-term tests lies in their ability to identify chemicals that may cause cancer under certain exposure conditions. More than 200 *in vitro* and *in vivo* short-term assays have been developed using bacteria, yeast, cultured mammalian cells and insects as testers. Most of the testers are engineered to detect one genetic end-point, such as mutations, deletions, genome rearrangements, loss of chromosomal fragment or whole chromosome. Tester strains were also constructed for simultaneous detection of several end-points. Typical example is the *Saccharomyces cerevisiae* D7 tester strain (Zimmermann et al. 1975) for detection of mitotic crossingover, gene conversion and reverse mutation. The current status of short-term tests for evaluation of genotoxicity, mutagenicity and carcinogenicity of chemicals and environmental pollutants has been recently reviewed (Bajpayee et al. 2005).

Generally, the short-term tests are rapid, inexpensive and easy to perform: results from bacterial tests are obtained in 3-4 days, and mammalian cell based assays are accomplished in about 10 days. Some bacterial cell-based assays are commercially available with results obtained in few hours. However, the advantage of having a fast procedure is compensated by the high unspecificity of the positive response: these tests detect all kind of DNA-damaging agents. Together with the possibility to analyze several samples simultaneously, these mentioned characteristics seem to be the main advantage of short-term tests. The mouse lymphoma assay and Chinese hamster ovary assay (Clive et al. 1979; Li et al. 1987) can detects genetic damages in viable cells capable of forming colonies, which permits the automatization of the methods. Cultured mammalian cells (*in vitro*) or bone marrow cells of rodents (*in vivo*) have been developed to study clastogenic response by analyses of chromosomal aberrations in metaphase cells or micronucleus formation. The micronucleus test (Neri et al. 2003) can be used along with kinetochore and centromeric staining to categorize the test compound as a clastogen or aneugen (Parry et al. 2002). Recently, the single cell gel electrophoresis (comet) assay gained popularity due to its rapidity and low cost (Singh et al. 1991). This assay can be performed both *in vivo* and *in vitro* to detect substantial DNA damages leading to fragmentation of the target DNA.

A significant advance was the development of cell transformation assays for a specific detection of carcinogens or to study the process of neoplastic transformation. The Syrian hamster embryo cell system (Le Boeuf et al, 1999) detects carcinogens within 10 days and has the advantage to be the only transformation system that employs normal diploid cells capable of metabolizing a wide spectrum of pro-carcinogens to their active form. The BALB/c3T3 mice cell system is based on a spontaneously immortalized cell line showing high sensitivity to transformation. Improvements of the assay showed a concordance of 73.5% with long-term bioassay (Kajiwara et al., 1997).

In conclusion, results from several appropriately selected short-term tests is now considered equivalent to the predictive value of a long-term bioassay. Short-term tests not only save time and expenses but also cut down the animal experimentation.

1.2 Disadvantages of short-term tests

The results of collaborative studies and the data accumulated, evidence that at present no single short-term assay can detect all genotoxic substances and discriminate noncarcinogenic mutagens from carcinogens. It is now accepted that batteries of tests have to be used in the study of mutagenic and/or carcinogenic properties of each potential genotoxin. Recommendations were made for strategies in testing which include several stages (usually three), each one consisting of 2 to 4 different assays and some of the tests (like the *Salmonella* mutagenicity test) have to be performed with 3-5 tester strains (Bajpayee et al. 2005; Eastmond et al. 2009). The necessity to perform a number of assays depreciates the main advantage of short-term tests - their rapidity and low cost. Short-term assays are used to study toxicity, mutagenicity and carcinogenicity of substances, however, the deep concern in such studies is mainly the presence of carcinogenic properties in pesticides, drugs, industrial wastages as well as pollutants of environment. Therefore, the need of having a short-term test for detection of carcinogenic activity in the start of testing for chemical risk assessment still exists. The cell transformation assays use the induction of certain phenotypic alterations that are related directly to neoplasia. The disadvantages of the assays seem to be the instability of the cell cultures used. Special precautions should be made to avoid culture and cell variations from different embryos and to maintain cells with the original karyotype. Therefore, the cell transformation assays can be successfully performed only in specialized laboratories by well trained personnel.

The *in vitro* mammalian cell assays detect a number of DNA damages in well characterized genes used as markers. However a correlation between the positive results and carcinogenicity is not always foolproof. There is increasing evidence that carcinogens acting through nongenotoxic mechanisms are not detected in these assays (Bajpayee et al. 2005). The interpretation of results from other assays may be also difficult. Thus, the chromosomal aberration *in vitro* assay is affected by artifacts due to cytotoxic doses of the studied compound, extreme pH values and metabolic activation that give false-positive results (Galloway 2000; Scott et al. 1991). The *in vivo* chromosomal aberration assay (Johnson et al. 1998) is used mainly for diagnosis, development and spread of tumors, rather than for screening studies (Szeles 2002). False-positive results can also be obtained with sister chromatide exchange measuring assays, since the majority of them do not represent genuine mutational events and are due to exchanges occurring in nonhomologous loci (Rodriguez-Reyes & Morales-Ramirez 2003).

The induction of micronuclei is related to dysfunction of spindle apparatus or formation of acentric fragments. Carcinogens give rise to these lesions during G1 to S phase transition of the cell cycle. The formation of micronuclei takes place in subsequent cell cycles and therefore one cell cycle is allowed between treatment and harvesting of cells. At shorter sample intervals micronuclei are not detected and at longer sampling time micronuclei are diluted and difficult for detection. Thus, results in the micronucleus test are greatly influenced by the time of treatment and sampling in relation to the cell cycle.

Some disadvantages of the comet assay have also been found. The main are: variations of results obtained because of the small cell sample, rate limiting of results due to the analysis of single cells, different interpretation of results due to variability in technical performance and cells utilized. Beside, the comet assay detects significant damages that result in DNA fragmentation and degradation usually associated with cell death (Split & Hartmann, 2005). Therefore this assay is less suitable for monitoring mutagenicity and clastogenicity of genotoxins.

In conclusion, most of the short-term tests have one genetic end-point associated with the activity of some, but not all carcinogens in the multistage process of differentiation the normal into malignant cells. Because of this, no one short-term test can detect all carcinogens and the usage of batteries of assays is recommended, which compromises the main advantage of the short-term assays - their rapidity and low cost. The few short-term tests having the process of neoplastic differentiation as an end-point are high tech methods requiring well equipped and specialized laboratories.

2. The Ty1 retrotransposon of *saccharomyces cerevisiae* is very similar to oncogenic retroviruses

Transposons are mobile DNA elements that replicate independently of the cellular genome and transpose the new copy into different places of nuclear DNA by nonhomologous recombination. They are ubiquitous from bacteria to human cells with a clear tendency to increase their copy number in higher eukaryotes: 45% of human DNA represents transposons and their remnants. Mobile elements that transpose to new sites in the genome via RNA intermediate are called retrotransposons because in many aspects they are analogous to the retroviruses, such as equine anemia virus, human immunodeficiency virus type 1 (HIV-1), yeast Ty1 transposon ect. (Garfinkel et al. 2006). Retroelements have been extensively studied in the yeast *S. cerevisiae*. Five distinct families of retrotransposons exists in this organism, named Ty1 to Ty5. Ty1 elements are the most abundant (33 copies per haploid genome), most highly expressed and most transpositionally active.

The structures of Ty1 retrotransposons and oncogenic retroviruses are very similar and consist of long terminal repeats (LTR) flanking a central coding domain including *gag* and *pol* genes (Figure 1). In the case of infectious retroviruses, an *env* gene is also present. The *gag* gene encodes structural proteins that form the retrotransposon virus-like particles (VLP), or the retroviral core particles, while the *pol* gene encodes the enzymes protease (PR), reverse transcriptase (RT) and integrase (IN). LTR retrotransposons and retroviruses are transcribed by RNA polymerase II from LTR to LTR to form a terminally redundant RNA molecule which is translated and packaged into the virion core particle or VLP.

Translation of Ty1 mRNA initiates close to its 5'end (Figure1). Like retroviruses, Ty1 elements employ translational frameshifting at the beginning of *pol* gene to regulate the expression of *gag* and *pol* gene products. The two open reading frames are overlapping and separated by a +1 frameshift occurring within a highly conserved sequence. The primary translation products are Gag-p49 and GagPol-p199 that are cleaved by PR to form mature Gag-p45, PR-p20, IN-p71 and RT-p63. The endogenous protease PR of Ty1 and retroviruses employs an aspartic residue in its catalytic centre. Finally, the processed subunits are assembled in VLPs where Ty1mRNA is used by RT as a template to generate double stranded Ty1 copyDNA that can be integrated by IN at new sites within the genome. The integration of the new Ty1 copy is often accompanied by the appearance of mutations, deletions, insertions, gene conversions, inversions or large genome rearrangements which labilize the structure of the host genome and may cause partial or complete loss of chromosomes (Garfinkel 2005). It should be noted that similar labilization of genome structure accompanied with chromosome loss occurred frequently during neoplastic differentiation of mammalian cells (Jeronimo et al. 2001).

The analysis of large variety of target sites has shown that 5' flanking regions of tRNA genes are the preferred target sites for Ty1 transposition (Mewes et al. 1997). Since the upstream regions of tRNA genes do not contain any special DNA sequences, the region-specific integration may be due to specific interactions of Ty1 integrase with the genome structure formed over the promoter elements of the tRNA gene (Nyswaner et al. 2008). Thus, Ty1 integration does not involve specific nucleotide sequence but a particular chromatine structure has the dominant role.

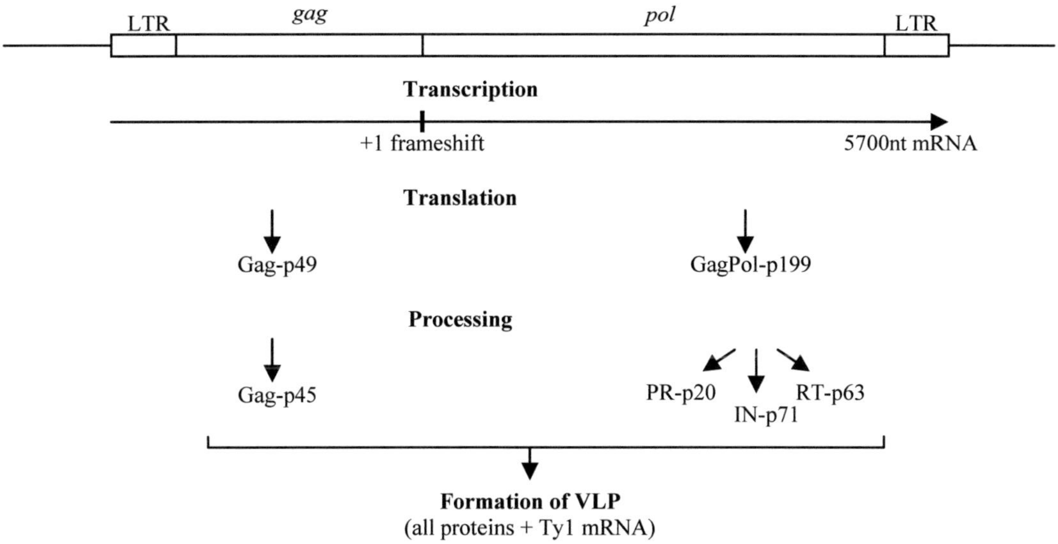

Fig. 1. Expression of Ty1 retrotransposon

Despite the high levels of Ty1 mRNA, transposition occurs at low level (10^{-5}-10^{-7}/cell/generation), cells contain low amount of mature Ty1 proteins and few VLPs are present. The balance needed between the level of *de novo* transposition and the Ty1 activity that can be tolerated by host yeast cell is reached by (1) a mechanism of transposition to specific target sites (upstream of tRNA genes), which are less hazardous for the cell because are devoid of protein coding function and, (2) regulatory mechanisms, that restrict Ty1 transposition to a low level. Both of these mechanisms lead to a decrease of successful Ty1 transpositions, thus saving the host from dangerous damages of DNA that may appear in the target site and result in labilizing the integrity of the genome.

The mobility of Ty1 retrotransposons is restricted by a large collection of proteins that preserve the integrity of the genome. Most of these repressors of transposition (Rtt) are ortologs of mammalian retroviral restriction factors (Curcio et al. 2007). The Rtt integrity factors inhibit transposition at posttranscriptional steps resulting in low level of Ty1 copyDNA. Two checkpoint pathways, the replication stress pathway and the DNA damage pathway, are involved in this type of Ty1 regulation in a cell-cycle dependent manner. Earlier studies (Staleva & Venkov 2001) also evidenced the dependence of Ty1 transposition upon transit through the cell cycle and *RAD9* gene product, which is a member of DNA damage signal transduction pathway. The protein product of *RAD9* checkpoint gene is the yeast functional counterpart of the human oncogene suppressor protein p53, which has among its functions monitoring the integrity of the genome and the delay of DNA replication until repair has been completed (Bertram 2001). These data suggest the existence of similarities in certain steps in regulation of Ty1 transposition and the neoplastic cells.

The analogy between Ty1 retrotransposons and retroviruses was recently confirmed in studies dealing with details in the mechanisms of their replication. The human APOBEC3G protein is similar to the APOBEC proteins of other eukaryotes and has been shown to inhibit the replication of Ty1 retrotransposon and retrooncoviruses. In all studied retroelements this inhibition represents a deamination of cytosines to uracils in copyDNA, which leads to degradation of the retroelement genome. An absolute requirement for a glutamate (E250Q) in the catalytic center of the different APOBEC proteins was found evidencing that DNA cytosine deamination is part of a mechanism, that restricts successful replication of Ty1 retrotransposons and retroviruses (Schumacher et al., 2008).

The surprising similarities between Ty1 retroelements and retroviruses become more understandable by the results obtained in phylogenetic studies (Llorens et al. 2009). The usage of combined graph and phylogenetic analysis based on genome sequencing data made possible the evolutionary history of LTR retroelements to be traced as a time-evolving network. The results obtained show that the Ty1 family represents the oldest pattern in this network and that diverse retroviruses evolve from LTR retrotransposons.

Mobile elements has a significant influence on evolution. Sequencing of diverse genomes reveals, that about half the spontaneous mutations in *Drosophila* result from insertions of mobile elements. In mammals mobile elements cause a smaller proportion of spontaneous mutations - 10% in mice and 0.2% in humans. It is presumed that mobile genetic elements have contributed to the evolution by promoting the creation of new genes with mutations favoring the adaptation (Garfinkel 2005). Thus, mobile genetic elements are probably one of the most powerful endogenous factors driving the evolution of all forms of life on earth.

In conclusion: according to genome structure, gene expression, life cycle, regulation of gene expression and evolutionary history, Ty1 retrotransposons are very similar to the oncogenic retroviruses, except for the absence of an infectious extracellular phase in their life cycle.

3. The Ty1 transposition test

Stress conditions, such as exposure to UV light (Rolfe & Banks 1986), low temperature treatment (Paquin & Williams 1984; Stamenova et al. 2008), severe adenine starvation (Ribero-dos-Santos et al. 1997) increase Ty1 transposition frequency. Chemical carcinogens can also increase transposition rate (Bradshow & McEntee 1989; Staleva & Venkov 2001). This, and the similarity in structure, gene expression and regulation reaching full analogy at certain points between Ty1 retrotransposons and oncogenic retroviruses suggested that the carcinogen-induced Ty1 transposition may be used for detection of carcinogenic genotoxins and substantiated the development of the Ty1 short-term test.

3.1 Construction of the tester strain

Two features have been considered important in the construction of the tester strain: (1) easy phenotypic detection of retrotransposition events and (2) increased permeability of tester yeast cells to carcinogens.

The indicator gene *HIS3AI* developed by Curcio & Garfinkel (1991) fulfills the first requirement. This reporter gene represents the *S. cerevisiae HIS3* gene interrupted by an artificial intron (AI) in the antisense orientation. The *HIS3AI* construction was inserted into a

Ty1 element with the intron on the sense strand of Ty1 and the marked Ty1 retrotransposon is integrated into the genome of a *S. cerevisiae* strain with deleted *HIS3* gene (Curcio & Garfinkel 1991). Thus, a successful transposition of the marked Ty1 element requires transcription, splicing the artificial intron, encapsulation in VLPs where Ty1 mRNA is reverse transcribed to give Ty1 copyDNA with functional *HIS3* gene. Every integration of this Ty1 copyDNA gives rise to one His$^+$ colony on selective medium lacking histidine. In contrast to other methods for determination of Ty1 transposition only in specific target loci (Ribeiro-dos-Santos et al., 1997), the usage of *HIS3AI* indicator gene permits tracing the Ty1 transposition in the genome as a whole. Another advantage of *HIS3AI* construction is that it allows direct selection of Ty1 transposition events in a single-step test. Since the number of His$^+$ transposants correlates directly with the number of transposition events for the marked Ty1 element, the usage of *HIS3AI* construction allows a *quantitative* determination of the transposition events. We used *HIS3AI* indicator gene for constructing the tester strain of Ty1 short-term test.

Yeast cells have been used to develop a variety of systems monitoring mutagens and carcinogens. Few of these tests, however, have an application in laboratory or environmental studies. The main reason seems to be the lower response of yeast cells as an indicator organism, due to limited uptake of genotoxins (Parry 1976), because of low permeability of *S. cerevisiae* cells (Morita et al. 1989). We overcome the natural inertness of yeast cells to mutagens and carcinogens by constructing a tester strain with increased cellular permeability. Previous studies revealed that a temperature-sensitive mutation, initially designated *ts1*, causes an increased cellular permeability of *S. cerevisiae* to different substances, including mutagens and carcinogens (Staleva et al. 1996). Cloning and sequencing showed that the *TS1* gene is the previously isolated *SEC53* gene and the *ts1/sec53* mutant allele represents a change of CCA to CTA (proline to leucine) at the 5′end of the gene (Staleva 1998). The essential *SEC53* gene codes for phosphomannomutase required in an early step in the pathway of O- and N-linked mannosylation (Kepes & Schekman 1988). Since the permeability barrier of *S. cerevisiae* is determined by the most superficial layer of the cell wall composed of highly glycosylated mannoproteins (Zlotnik et al. 1989), the impairment of protein glycosylation in *sec53* mutant cells results in formation of a permeability barrier with insufficient functions.

Strain	Cell wall porosity after cultivation at:			
	23°C		30°C	
550 (*SEC53*)	25.58 ± 3.47		23.96 ± 4.86	
551 (*sec53*)	29.25 ± 5.83		93.85 ± 7.22	
	Transformation with plasmid DNA (transformants per 1μg DNA)			
	+LiAc		-LiAc	
	23°C	30°C	23°C	30°C
550 (*SEC53*)	1820 ± 43	2024 ± 18	0	0
551 (*sec53*)	1682 ± 67	2120 ± 31	2 ± 1	172 ± 44

LiAc -Lithium Acetate

Table 1. Increased permeability of *S. cerevisiae* 551 cells LiAc -Lithium Acetate.

Average values ± SD of 6 experiments. The porosity of cell wall was calculated as percentages following the recommendations of the authors (DeNobel & Barnett, 1991). The transformation procedure (Ito et al., 1983) with YCP50 plasmid DNA was used to obtain Ura^+ transformants.

The replacement of *SEC53* gene in the tester strain with the *sec53* mutant allele was performed by means of the two-step gene replacement method (Sherman et al. 2001). Briefly, the *sec53* allele was cloned in an integrative *URA3*-marked vector, restricted in the unique AlfII site of the *SEC53* gene and tester cells were transformed to give Ura^+ integrative transformants. Strains having the *sec53* allele instead of the *SEC53* wild type gene were selected (Pesheva et al. 2005), one of the selected transformants was named *S. cerevisiae* 551 and used as a tester strain in the Ty1 assay. Its genotype is: *MATa ura3 his3Δ200 TymHIS3AI sec53, rho*$^+$. The *S. cerevisiae* 551 strain is deposited with №8719 into the National Bank for Industrial Microorganisms and Cell Cultures (Sofia, Bulgaria).

The temperature of 37°C is nonpermissive for both, Ty1 transposition (Paquin & Williams, 1984) and the growth of cells having the *sec53* temperature sensitive mutant allele. Cultivated at the semirestrictive temperature of 30°C, tester cells are growing exponentially with generation time of about 150 min in YEPD liquid medium and partial expression of the *sec53* phenotype. Significantly lower survival rates due to increased uptake of genotoxic substances were obtained for *S. cerevisiae* 551 cells grown at 30°C and treated with a variety of genotoxins compared to the isogenic *SEC53* harboring cells at equal concentrations of the chemicals. Direct evidence for increased permeability of yeast cells were obtained using the porosity test (DeNobel & Barnett 1991) and the transformation procedure with plasmid DNA (Ito et al., 1983). A fourfold increase in porosity was found only for *S. cerevisiae* 551 cells cultivated at 30°C (Table1). The porosity of the isogenic *S. cerevisiae* 550 cells (having the wild type *SEC53* gene) remained identical after cultivation at 23°C or 30°C. The increased permeability of *S. cerevisiae* 551 cells was also confirmed by their transformability with plasmid DNA. Wild type yeast cells are not permeable for plasmid DNA and in order to be transformed, the permeability of intact *S. cerevisiae* cells is increased by treatment with lithium acetate (Ito et al. 1983) or the cells are converted to spheroplasts. We obtained relatively high frequency of transformation (5-6%) for intact 551 cells grown at 30°C and not treated with lithium acetate (Pesheva et al. 2005). Transformants were not obtained from 550 cells without lithium acetate treatment either at 23°C or at 30°C, as expected. All these results evidence an increased cellular permeability of *S. cerevisiae* 551 cells at 30°C due to the *sec53* mutation and supported the usage of *S. cerevisiae* 551 as a tester strain in the Ty1 short-term assay.

3.2 The Ty1 transposition test: A laboratory protocol

1. *S. cerevisiae* 551 cells are cultivated at 30°C in water bath shaker in YEPD liquid medium (the recipes of used media are given in Sherman et al. 2001) to a density of 5-7x10^7cells/ml.
2. The culture is divided into samples of 4ml and appropriate concentrations of the studied genotoxins added. Water insoluble substances are dissolved in dimethylsulfoxide (Me_2SO) or ethanol and used in volumes not exceeding a final concentration of 5% of Me_2SO or ethanol. The control samples are treated with the same volume of the solvent.

3. Samples are cultivated at 30°C for 30 min in water bath shaker; cells are washed with YEPD liquid medium by centrifugation and suspended in 4ml fresh YEPD medium.
4. Cells are cultivated at 20°C in water bath shaker for 24h to complete initiated Ty1 transposition events. As it will be shown later on the cultivation at 20°C results in about 5 fold higher rate of successful transpositions relative to cultivation at 30°C.
5. Appropriate dilutions (usually 10^{-4}-10^{-5}) are made in sterile water and 0.1ml is plated on each YEPD plate. Use at least five YEPD plates to determine cell titer of survivals for control and for each concentration of the genotoxin.
6. The remaining part of each sample is centrifuged; cells are washed twice with sterile water and suspended in 3.9ml of water. Ten SC-His plates are plated with 0.2ml suspension per plate to determine the number of His^+ transformants for controls and for each concentration of the genotoxin.
7. Plates are incubated at 30°C for 3 days (YEPD plates) or 5 days (SC-His plates) and colonies are counted.
8. Median transposition rates are determined by the equation:

Fold Increase = Fts/Ftc, where

$$Fts = \frac{Number\ of\ His + transposans\ of\ treated\ culture}{Number\ of\ survivors\ devided\ by\ fold\ dilution\ of\ treated\ culture}$$

$$Ftc = \frac{Number\ of\ His + transposans\ of\ control\ culture}{Number\ of\ survivors\ devided\ by\ fold\ dilution\ of\ control\ culture}$$

Results can also be presented as "fold increase" of Ty1 transposition rates relative to the rate of transposition in the control sample taken as a fold increase of 1.0. A fold increase equal or higher than 2.0 is considered as a positive response of the Ty1 short-term test.

Note: When metabolic activation is needed to convert pre-mutagens and pre-carcinogens to their active forms, S9 mix is added to samples 60 min before the treatment with genotoxins. *S. cerevisiae* cells have cytochrom P_{450} and P_{488} required for the metabolic activation of pre-genotoxins. The activation of this intrinsic metabolic system can be achieved by switching cells growing in low dextrose (0.2%) to high dextrose (10%) YEPD liquid medium (Kelly & Perry 1983). After 3-4 generations in the high dextrose medium cells can be used in the Ty1 test without addition of an exogenous S9 mix and the presence of S9 mix does not change the results obtained. The change from low to high dextrose medium is made in a very early exponential growth phase (about $2x10^7$cells/ml) to allow for several generations before the treatment with pre-genotoxins.

4. Response of Ty1 test to laboratory genotoxins

Laboratory genotoxins with different structure and mode of action have been used to study the main characteristics of the Ty1 short-term test.

4.1 Increased sensitivity of Ty1 test

Benzo(a)pyrene [B(a)P] although being a very active agent in the *Salmonella* system, does not induce genetic damages in wild type *S. cerevisiae,* because little of this aromatic compound is taken up by yeasts due to the limited permeability of cells. The results obtained in the Ty1 test (Table 2) show that this is true when *S. cerevisiae* 550 cells with wild type of *SEC53* gene are used as testers. However, if *S. cerevisiae* 551 (*sec53*) strain was used, the Ty1 test responds to increased concentrations of B(a)P with enhanced rate of Ty1 transposition. The positive answer of the test appears at low concentrations of B(a)P having negligible effect on cell - survival and the fold increase of Ty1 transposition rates enhanced in a concentration dependent manner.

Strain	B(a)P (mM)	S9 mix	Survival (%)	Ty1 test (fold increase)	$O_2^{-\cdot}$ (pM/cell)[a)]
551 (*sec53*)	0	-	100	1.00	0.048
	0	+	100	1.00	0.054
	0.08	-	105	0.71	0.045
	0.08	+	91	4.87	0.581
	0.16	-	85	1.41	0.080
	0.16	+	80	9.18	1.221
	0.32	-	63	2.00	0.080
	0.32	+	56	18.41	2.450
551+NaN_2[b)]	0.15	-	38	1.22	0.063
550 (*SEC53*)	0	-	100	1.00	0.040
	0	+	100	1.00	0.045
	0.08	-	98	1.27	0.061
	0.08	+	102	1.18	0.082
	0.16	-	105	1.85	0.062
	0.16	+	95	2.00	0.079
	0.32	-	88	1.67	0.055
	0.32	+	82	2.50	0.121
550+NaN_2[b)]	0.15	-	52	1.25	0.068

Typical results from one out of six identical experiments

[a)] Amount of superoxide anion ($O_2^{-\cdot}$) in pM per one cell determined by the method described in Stamenova et al. (2008)

[b)] Cells treated only with NaN_2

Table 2. Increased sensitivity of Ty1 test to metabolically activated B(a)P

Similar increase in the values of Ty1 transposition rates was also found in kinetic experiments where cells were treated for periods of 15 to 90 minutes. The positive answer of Ty1 test is not due to the stress conditions generated by the increased cellular toxicity at higher concentrations of B(a)P, since treatment with NaN_3, a powerful cell poison, had no effect on Ty1 transposition. Similar positive responses of the Ty1 test were found in concentration dependent and kinetic experiments with a number of carcinogenic genotoxins showing low response in tests based on wild type of yeast cells (Dimitrov et al., 2011; Pesheva et al., 2005; 2008; Staleva & Venkov 2001).

4.2 The Ty1 test responds positively only to active carcinogens

B(a)P is a pre-carcinogen which has to be metabolically activated in order to produce its effect in the cell. The Ty1 test used with the highly permeable 551 strain as tester cells did not respond positively after treatment with B(a)P in absence of S9 mix (Table 2). The percentage of cells that survived this treatment decreases with increasing B(a)P concentration suggesting that ones inside cells the pre-carcinogen has a toxic effect which however is not an inducer of Ty1 transposition. The Ty1 test was positive with B(a)P and different other pre-carcinogens only in presence of S9 metabolizing mix (Dimitrov et al. 2011; Pesheva et al. 2005; 2008). These results evidence that the *sec53* mutation in *S. cerevisiae* 551 tester strain increases the sensitivity of Ty1 test due to increased permeability of cells. In addition, the positive response of the test to active carcinogens and the negative results obtained with pre-carcinogens suggest a specificity of the test response to the active forms of the genotoxins.

4.3 The Ty1 test is positive with carcinogens not detectable in the other short-term tests

Every short-term test has a range of carcinogen's detection and the usage of batteries of tests extends the limits of detection. Nevertheless, a fraction of genotoxins with carcinogenic potential proved in long-term experiments did not induce any short-term assay tested up to the maximum solubility and the reasons for this are not known (Ramel et al. 1996). We studied representatives of these genotoxins in the Ty1 test and results are summarized in Table 3.

Carcinogen	Concentration (mM)	Survival (%)	Ty1 transposants per/10^8cells	Ty1 test (fold increase)	$O_2^{\cdot-}$ (pM/cell)
Control	-	100	25 ± 5	1.0	0.045±0.001
Carcinogens negative in Salmonella tests					
Acetamide	34	60	172 ± 18	7.82	0.284±0.041
Thioacet-amide	13	71	182 ± 24	8.23	0.315±0.048
Dichloro-methane	10	58	193 ± 31	8.76	0.421±0.055
Carcinogens negative in all short-term tests					
Furfuryl alcohol	5	45	110 ± 8	5.0	0.470±0.028
Tetrahydro-furan	5	58	121 ± 12	5.5	0.520±0.055
tert-butyl-hydroquinone	0.05	53	134 ± 16	6.1	1.020±0.099
Noncarcinogenic mutagens					
5-bromuracil	52	50	33 ± 4	1.5	0.050±0.015
Benzo(e) pyrene[a)]	160	61	41 ± 6	1.9	0.068±0.005
Anthracene[a)]	34	72	26 ± 7	1.2	0.048±0.010

Average values ± SD of 5 experiments

[a)]Benzo(e)pyrene and anthracene were dissolved in Me_2SO and tested in presence of S9 mix of Ty1 test did not result from secondary effects of dying cells and the test responds positively to some carcinogens not detectable by the other short-term assays.

Table 3. Wider range of Ty1 test in carcinogen's detection

Furfuryl alcohol, tetrahydrofuran and *tert*-butylhydroquinone which are carcinogens not detectable in the other short-term tests showed a positive response in Ty1 test (Dimitrov et al., 2011;Pesheva et al. 2005). With increasing the time of exposure (15 to 45 min) the frequency of Ty1 transposition steadily increased and reached a plateau suggesting saturation of transposition rates. After 30 min exposure to different concentrations, the tester cells exhibited a dose response with an increase at higher concentrations of the carcinogens. The induction of Ty1 transposition (fold increase >2.0) started before significant cell death become apparent. Based on these data, it is concluded that the carcinogen-stimulated positive response to some carcinogens not detectable by the other short term assays.

Negative results in Ty1 test were obtained with 5-bromuracil, anthracene and benzo(e)pyrene [B(e)P] which are mutagens without carcinogenic potential (Table 3). The positive results in Ty1 test found for a number of carcinogens, the specific test response to only metabolically activated carcinogens and the absence of response to noncarcinogenic mutagens suggested that Ty1 test may have the ability to differentiate carcinogens from mutagens without carcinogenic properties.

Genotoxin	Concentration [a)] (mM)	Survival (%)	Ty1 test (fold increase)	$O_2^{.-}$ (pM/cell)
Controls				
H_2O	-	100	1.0	0.048±0.009
Me_2SO	5%	98	1.1	0.058±0.010
Carcinogens				
B(a)A	26	57	14.5	2.450±0.205
CDH	1000	48	16.0	2.851±0.221
LH	1000	53	22.0	3.446±0.255
CrVI	5	54	47.3	4.405±0.366
Noncarcinogenic mutagens				
B(b)A	26	70	1.8	0.068±0.005
TDH	1000	61	1.8	0.045±0.009
GDH	1000	80	1.5	0.058±0.010
CrIII	5	59	1.3	0.031±0.005

Average values of 6 experiments
Me_2SO - dimettylsulfoxide; B(a)A - benzo(a)anthracene; B(b)A- benzo(b)anthracene; CrVI - hexavalent chromium; CrIII - trivalent chromium; CDH - chenodeoxycholic bile acid; LH - lithocholic bile acid; TDH - taurodeoxycholic bile acid; GDH- glycodeoxycholic bile acid
[a)]CrVI and CrIII were dissolved in water; all the other genotoxins were dissolved in Me_2SO and tested in the presence of S9 mix

Table 4. Selective response of Ty1 test to carcinogens

4.4 Selective response of Ty1 test to carcinogens

The possibility that Ty1 test may have a selective positive response to carcinogens was studied using pairs of genotoxins with close to identical chemical structure: the one being strong carcinogen and the second having only mutagenic properties without being a carcinogen. One such pair is the well known carcinogen B(a)P and the B(e)P which is a noncarcinogenic mutagen. The carcinogenic status of all compounds used in our studies was according to YARC (1990) and recent publications in the field (Donkin et al. 2000). As it was already shown (Tables 2, 3) B(a)P induces strong positive answer in Ty1 test, while B(e)P was without effect on Ty1 transposition rate.

Benzo(a)anthracene [B(a)A] and benzo(b)anthracene [B(b)A] represent another pair of genotoxins studied in the Ty1 test (Dimitrov et al.,2011; Pesheva et al. 2008). B(a)A is assessed as carcinogenic for animals and humans while B(b)A is a non-carcinogenic mutagen (Salamone 1981). The study of these genotoxins in the Ty1 test (Table 4) showed a strong positive answer for the carcinogenic B(a)A and negative result (fold increase < 2.0) for the noncarcinogenic mutagen B(b)A. Table 4 shows results obtained at equimolar concentrations and the absence of positive test-response was also found for higher concentrations of B(b)A killing up to 70% of tester cells.

Considerable evidence support the view that free, but not conjugated, bile acids are carcinogenic in humans (reviewed in Bernstein et al. 2005). We took advantage from these observations to further characterize Ty1 test and studied the effect of the free chenodeoxycholic (CDH) and lithocholic (LH) bile acids and the noncarcinogenic conjugated taurodeoxycholic (TDH) and glycodeoxycholic (GDH) bile acids (Pesheva et al. 2008). The results obtained (Table 4) show that the carcinogenic CDH and LH bile acids induced positive responses in the Ty1 test, whereas the noncarcinogenic TDH and GDH bile acids give values close to the controls. While the two free bile acids increase the frequency of Ty1 transposition over a tenfold concentration range, the conjugated acids showed no such activity, even though toxicities of up to 60% were produced.

Although some heavy metals (the so-called trace elements) are essential for the survival of all life forms, others can be quite toxic and carcinogenic. In preliminary experiments we studied the response of Ty1 test to arsenic (As) classified as confirmed human carcinogen, lead (Pb) categorized as probable human carcinogen and zinc (Zn) which is not classifiable with regard to human carcinogenicity (Dimitrov et al. 2011). The results obtained were positive for As and Pb in concentration and time dependent experiments, while Zn was without effect on Ty1 transposition. A special interest represents the pair hexavalent chromium (CrVI) and trivalent chromium (CrIII). While CrVI is confirmed as strong human carcinogen, the data for CrIII are controversial. An extensive recent review (Eastmond et al. 2008) points to many instances of conflicting information. Thus, *in vitro* data suggest that CrIII has the potential to react with DNA and to cause DNA damages which however required experimental conditions incompatible with cell-life. *In vivo* evidence suggest that genotoxic effects did not occur in human cells or animals exposed to CrIII and the trivalent chromium complexes are widely used for decades as nutritional supplements and insulin enhancers in patients with type 2 diabetes. Although firm data for a carcinogenic effect of CrIII are lacking, there is a growing concern (Levina & Lay 2008) over a possible carcinogenicity of CrIII based on the assumption that once in the cell, part of CrIII can be oxidized to CrVI which is a confirmed human carcinogen. The study of CrVI and CrIII in the Ty1 test confirmed the strong carcinogenic effect of CrVI with a fold increase of 47 following treatment with 5mM CrVI for 30 min (Table 4). At the same conditions CrIII gave values close to the controls, as did all studied till now noncarcinogenic mutagens. Regardless of results that will be obtained in the future in favor of presence or absence of carcinogenicity for CrIII, it should be noted that the data obtained with CrVI and CrIII evidence that the Ty1 short-term test possesses the characteristic to discriminate opposite effects of a heavy metal, determined by changes in its valence.

5. Response of Ty1 test to environmental pollutants

Biomonitoring requires accurate, sensitive, easy and fast methods to assay environmental pollution. The specific and selective response of Ty1 short-term test to carcinogens found with laboratory genotoxins suggested a verification of the characteristics of the assay in environmental studies monitoring pollution. The study was conducted during 2006-2007 and consisted of monitoring pollution in soil, water and air in regions in Bulgaria (Pesheva et al. 2008), using Ty1 test and quantitative chemical analysis of the samples. Processed samples were chemically analyzed for presence of mutagens, carcinogens, pesticides, polychlorinated biophenols, heavy metals, etc., at a total of 53 substances. In this review only short excerpts of the protocols will be presented, and, results obtained for air and water samples will be omitted.

Soil samples were collected from regions with low (odd number) or high (even number samples) pollution levels in June 2006 (S1, S2), November 2006 (S3, S4), May 2007 (S5, S6) and October 2007 (S8). Samples were processed according to standard procedures and each extract of sample was directly analyzed chemically and studied with Ty1 test in presence of S9 metabolic activating mix. Such experimental program gives the advantage to directly compare results obtained in the short-term test with the amount of genotoxins found in the chemically analysis of the samples. Samples collected from clean region showed low toxicity and gave negative responses in Ty1 test (Table 5). These results evidence that the Ty1 assay does not give false positives with extracts of samples. Samples collected from polluted regions showed different toxicities on yeast cells with a higher toxic effect of samples containing petrol products (S8). All samples from polluted regions gave positive results in Ty1 test with a fold increase ranging 7-12. The positive answers were confirmed in concentrations (= sample volume) dependent and kinetics experiments (Pesheva et al. 2008). The chemical analysis Table 5 shows that samples from the clean regions did not contain any carcinogenic genotoxins, while all samples from polluted regions contain mixtures of carcinogens. Only substances found in amounts above the accepted ecological standards are shown on (Table 5). Since each sample from polluted regions contained several carcinogenic substances, their positive results evidence that the Ty1 test responds positively to mixtures of carcinogens, as well.

Special attention should be given to samples S1 and S3 collected from clean regions which showed negative results in the Ty1 test. These samples were polluted with flouranthrene at concentrations 0.28 mg/kg and 0.19 mg/kg for S1 and S3, respectively. Given the accepted ecological maximum of 0.02 mg/kg, it is clear that although S1 and S3 samples are heavily polluted with flouranthrene they show negative results in Ty1 test. It has consistently been shown that fluoranthrene proved to be a potent mutagen in bacterial and mammalian *in vitro* test systems, however results from *in vivo* carcinogenicity studies in rodents evidenced it is not carcinogenic (Goldman et all. 2001; Verschueren 2001). Thus the selective response of Ty1 test to carcinogens found in studies with laboratory genotoxins is also characteristic for the assay used in environmental studies.

A short excerpt of the chemical analysis of soil samples is given in Table 6. For all mutagens and carcinogens that were analyzed but not included in the table, concentrations values below the accepted ecological standards were found. The results showed the significant pollution of samples collected from polluted regions. The amounts of some carcinogenic heavy metals (Pb, As, Cd) were 4-6 fold higher and the samples were polluted with mixtures of the carcinogenic genotoxins (B(a)P, B(a)A, benzo(hgi)pyrene, petrol products) and different mutagens.

Sample	Survival (%)	Ty1 transposants [a] (per 10^8 cells)	Ty1 test (fold increase)	Mutagens/carcinogens [b] found in chemical analysis
Control				
Me_2SO 5%	100	18 ± 5	1.0	
Clean Regions				
S1	92	22 ± 6	1.2	fluoranthrene
S3	90	27 ± 8	1.5	fluoranthrene
S5	97	31 ± 6	1.7	
Polluted regions				
S2	78	131 ± 16	7.3	**As**, **B(a)P**, **B(a)A**, **pyrene**, **crysene**, **benzo(ghi)perylene**, **Pb**, B(e)P, fluoranthrene
S4	67	127 ± 18	7.1	**As**, **B(a)P**, **pyrene**, **crysene**, **Pb**, B(e)P,
S6	79	99 ± 9	5.5	**As**, **B(a)P**, **pyrene**, **crysene**, **Pb**, fluoranthrene
S8	42	228 ± 21	12.7	**B(a)P**, **B(a)A**, **pyrene**, **crysene**, **petrol products**, **Pb**, B(e)P, B(b)A

[a] Average values ± SD from 10 experiments
[b] Carcinogenes are shown in bold

Table 5. Response of Ty1 test to soil samples

Carcinogens or mutagens	Ecological Standard (mg/kg)	Pollutants in soil samples (mg/kg)						
		Clean regions samples			Polluted regions samples			
		S1	S3	S5	S2	S4	S6	S8
Pb	50	31	24	29	364	386	348	287
As	25	15	9	12	113	93	82	199
Cd	2	0.4	0.3	0.5	2.2	3.2	1.5	1.8
Anthracene	0.05	0.00	0.01	0.02	0.04	0.06	0.02	0.09
Flouranthene	0.02	0.28	0.19	0.03	0.24	0.06	0.13	0.49
B(e)P	0.02	0.01	0.01	0.00	0.09	0.18	0.00	0.18
B(a)P	0.02	0.00	0.00	0.00	0.06	0.18	0.00	0.21
Benzo(ghi)pyrene	0.02	0.00	0.00	0.00	0.09	0.00	0.00	0.01
Petrol products	50	0.00	0.00	0.00	2	8	25	195
Pyrene	0.02	0.02	0.02	0.02	0.28	0.05	0.18	0.49
B(a)A	0.02	0.02	0.02	0.02	0.10	0.03	0.05	0.47
Chrysene	0.01	0.01	0.00	0.00	0.12	0.07	0.06	0.24

Table 6. Chemical analysis of soil samples

The samples collected from clean regions did not contain carcinogens above the ecological standards, although some of them (S1, S3) were polluted with flouranthene as already discussed. The analysis of environmental samples in Ty1 test permits an evaluation of the

Ty1 test sensitivity in environmental studies. An assay should be sensitive enough to detect levels of carcinogens over the accepted standards and to not give false positives with carcinogen's concentration below the ecological standards. The accepted standards for the different mutagenic or carcinogenic substances indicate the amounts of genotoxins that are not harmful for humans and animals. Table 6 (the three bottom lines) show that samples S1, S3, S5 contain pyrene at concentrations of 0.02 mg/kg which is the ecological standard. Samples S1 and S3 contain also B(a)A at concentrations close to the ecological standard and sample S1 contains 0.01 mg/kg of chrysene which is the accepted standard for this carcinogen. All these samples give negative results in Ty1 test (Table 5) evidencing that this assay remains negative with concentrations of carcinogens bellow the ecological standards. Together, the results obtained in environmental studies evidence that Ty1 test detects selectively carcinogenic pollutants only if they are in concentrations above the accepted ecological standards.

6. The molecular mechanism of the selective response to carcinogens

The positive and selective response to carcinogenic genotoxins requires explanation and two observations directed our efforts to clarify the molecular mechanism of the Ty1 test response.

First, we noted that the appearance of *rho*$^-$ mutants among His$^+$ transposants induced by carcinogens, is a very rare event. *S. cerevisiae rho*$^-$ cells are mitochondrial mutants representing large deletions of mitochondrial DNA (mtDNA), that appear spontaneously (Dujon, 1981), or can be induced by treatment with ethidium bromide (Sherman et al. 2001) or freezing (Stamenova et al. 2007). Nine out of ten studied carcinogens induced only *rho*$^+$ transposants (with wild type mtDNA) and the percentage of *rho*$^-$ transposants induced by *tert*-butylhydroquinoline was below the spontaneous frequency. This results and the observation that treatment with different carcinogens of *rho*$^-$ mutants was without effect on Ty1 transposition (Stoycheva et al. 2007; 2008), strongly suggested that the carcinogen induced positive response in Ty1 test depends on the function of mitochondria.

Although the deleted mtDNA fragment spans over different number of genes in *rho*$^-$ mutants, the genes for oxidative phosphorylation are deleted in all *rho*$^-$ isolates irrespective of the way they are induced (Dujon 1981). The nuclear gene *SCO1* codes for a protein that is transported to mitochondria where it participates in formation of oxidative phosphorylation complexes (Glerum et al. 1996). Mutations in, or disruption of the *SCO1* gene are associated with respiratory deficiency, however in contrast to *rho*$^-$ mutants, *sco1* mutants lack only mitochondrial oxidative phosphorylation in otherwise intact and functional mitochondria. We disrupted *SCO1* gene in *S. cerevisiae* 551 tester strain and the study of carcinogen-induced Ty1 transposition in 551 *sco1Δ* cells showed absence of Ty1 induction with almost equal Ty1 transposition rates in *sco1Δ*, *rho*$^-$ or control cells (Stoycheva et al. 2010). Therefore, the Ty1 transposition induced by carcinogens depends on oxidative phosphorylation and not on another mitochondrial function.

The second observation we made came from an extensive survey of the literature showing that all carcinogens with positive answer in Ty1 test are powerful generators of reactive oxygen species (ROS) in different cells (Bernstein et al. 2007; Toyooka & Ibuki 2007) including *S. cerevisiae* (Brennan & Schiestl 1998; Herrero et al. 2008). The data for noncarcinogenic mutagens, although not abundant, showed absence of, or negligible effect on cellular level of ROS (Scandalios 2005; Toyooka & Ibuki 2007). ROS are generated in aerobic organisms through both endogenous and exogenous routes. The majority of endogenous ROS are produced through leakage of superoxide anions ($O_2^{\cdot -}$) from the mitochondrial respiratory chain.

ROS are generated by one electron reduction of O_2 or formed from enzymatic systems (Fridovich 1997). Dismutation of $O_2^{\cdot -}$ (spontaneously or by superoxide dismutases) produces hydrogen peroxide (H_2O_2) which in the presence of metal ions is partially reduced to hydroxyl radical (·OH). To minimize the damaging effects of ROS, aerobic cells evolved nonenzymatic and enzymatic antioxidant defenses. At increased levels, however ROS can not be detoxified sufficiently and may have deleterious effects on lipids, fatty acids, proteins and DNA. A variety of DNA lesions, block of replication and chromosomal loss were frequently detected in cells under oxidative stress.

We studied the possible link between carcinogen-induced Ty1 transposition and ROS level by simultaneous determination of Ty1 mobility and $O_2^{\cdot -}$ levels following treatment with carcinogens. As shown on Tables 2, 3 and 4 (last columns) the treatment with carcinogens increased both, Ty1 transposition rate and $O_2^{\cdot -}$ in tester cells, while noncarcinogenic mutagens (Table 4) have little effect on Ty1 mobility and $O_2^{\cdot -}$ level. We used a method for quantitative determination of $O_2^{\cdot -}$ in live cells only (Stamenova et al. 2008), so that the various toxicities of genotoxins can not account for the different amount of $O_2^{\cdot -}$ found in cells treated with carcinogens or noncarcinogenic mutagens.

Strain	Temperature of cultivation (°C)	MMS (3.5mM)	Ty1 transposants (per 10^8 live cells)
551 *rho*⁻	15	-	72 ± 6
	30	-	16 ± 3
551 *rho*⁺	15	-	87 ± 7
	30	-	19 ± 6
551 *rho*⁻	15	+	78 ± 8
	30	+	17 ± 4
551 *rho*⁺	15	+	641 ± 32
	30	+	155 ± 18

Average values ±SD from 6 experiments

Table 7. Ty1 transposition at different temperatures

Another possible reason to fall into error studying the interactions between carcinogen-induced Ty1 transposition and ROS level would be that the whole process of transposition in *rho*⁻ cells is impeded from unknown yet reason and cells are unable to carry out Ty1 transposition at all. It has been shown that the rate of spontaneous transposition in cells cultivated at temperatures of 15°C increases relative to cells grown at 30°C (Paquin & Williamson 1984). We confirmed this result and as shown on Table 7 the number of *spontaneous* His⁺ transposants in *rho*⁻ cells at 15°C was significantly higher compared to cells grown at 30°C. However, treatment of *rho*⁻ cells with the carcinogen methylmethanesulfonate (MMS) did not enhance Ty1 transposition rates at any of the two temperatures. In *rho*$^+$ cells the increase of spontaneous and MMS-induced Ty1 transpositions was evident after cultivation at 15°C and 30°C. Since *rho*$^+$ and *rho*$^-$ cells increase spontaneous transposition rates at 15°C by an equal factor of 5 relative to cultivation at 30°C, the reason for absence of carcinogen-induced Ty1 transposition in *rho*$^-$ cells is not a general defect in the transposition process and most likely is due to loss of the start signal for the carcinogen induced transposition.

Several lines of evidence confirmed the role of increased ROS levels as inducers of Ty1 transposition in *S. cerevisiae* cells treated with carcinogens.

Although tightly coupled, the two processes in mitochondrial phosphorylation, electron transfer and ATP synthesis, can be selectively inhibited: antimycinA inhibits the transfer of electrons while carbonyl cyanide-3-chlorophenyl hydrazine (CCCP) blocks ATP synthesis (Epstein et al. 2001). Tester 551 cells cultivated in presence of antimycinA showed significant higher Ty1 transposition rates (fold increase 30-40) upon treatment with MMS compared to cells with not inhibited electron transfer and treated with the same concentration of MMS (fold increase 6-8). The block of ATP synthesis with CCCP had little or no effect on MMS-induced Ty1 mobility (Stoycheva et al. 2010). The inhibition of electron transfer along the respiratory chain is known to increase the leakage of electrons and to enhance in this way the production of ROS (Rasmussen et al., 2003). Higher ROS levels are also generated in exponential cells and cells growing in high dextrose (2%) media vs. stationary cells and cells cultivated in low dextrose (0.2%) media (Barros et al.,; 2004Lin et al., 2002). The study of MMS-induced Ty1 transposition showed increased mobility of Ty1 in exponential cells and cells from high dextrose medium compared to stationary cells and cells grown in low dextrose medium. The activation of Ty1 mobility by carcinogens seems to depend on accumulation of $O_2^{\cdot-}$ generated by the carcinogens since addition of N-acetylcysteine (NAC), a scavenger of $O_2^{\cdot-}$, resulted in absence of both, the increase in $O_2^{\cdot-}$ levels and the induction of Ty1 transposition rates (Table 8). The elevation of $O_2^{\cdot-}$ level with menadione, a superoxide generator, also increases Ty1 mobility without any additional treatment with carcinogen. Taken together, these results show that yeast cells with functioning oxidative phosphorylation accumulate $O_2^{\cdot-}$ upon treatment with carcinogens and indicate a key role of enhanced ROS levels in activating the initiation of the Ty1 transposition process.

S. cerevisiae has been shown to have distinct protective responses to superoxides and peroxides (Jamieson et al. 1992). The *YAP1* gene encodes a transcription factor that activates target genes involved in response against H_2O_2 (Nguyen et al. 2001) and mutants deleted for *YAP1* gene accumulate H_2O_2 in the cells. We disrupted the *YAP1* gene in 551 tester strain and found 551*yap1Δ* cells to respond upon carcinogen treatment with significantly higher induction of Ty1 mobility compared to cells with functioning *YAP1* gene. A dose-dependent increase of ROS following exposure of cells to exogenously added H_2O_2 was found in numerous studies (Tample et al. 2005 and citations therein). We used this observation to supply *rho*$^-$ cells with the missing ROS and studied Ty1 transposition in the 551 *rho*$^-$ strain treated with increased concentrations of H_2O_2. Treatment with 0.5, 1.0 and 3.0mM H_2O_2 induced Ty1 transposition with a fold increase of 6, 10 and 25, respectively, relative to the nontreated control.

Carcinogen (mM)	NAC[a)] (60mM)	MD[b)] (mM)	Survival (%)	$O_2^{\cdot-}$ (pM/cell)[c)]	Ty1 test (fold increase)
Control (H_2O)	-	-	100	0.045 ± 0.015	1.0
MMS (3.0)	-	-	45	0.387 ± 0.115	8.5
MMS (3.0)	+	-	78	0.040 ± 0.010	0.9
As (2.0)	-	-	51	0.871 ± 0.250	33.5
As (2.0)	+	-	82	0.053 ± 0.009	0.8
CrVI(5.0)	-	-	54	1.440 ± 0.410	41.3
CrVI(5.0)	+	-	75	0.048 ± 0.018	1.7
-	-	2	81	0.788 ± 0.115	4.5
-	-	5	41	2.675 ± 0.550	8.1

[a)] N-acetylcysteine added 1h before treatment with carcinogens
[b)] Menadione added for 1h
[c)] Average of 4 experiments

Table 8. Response of *S. cerevisiae* 551 cells to carcinogens depends on ROS level

In addition to the transposition process, the movement and integration of Ty1 transposon to a new location in the genome can also occur by gene conversion (Roeder & Fink 1982). In this process a resident Ty1 element without being replicated undergoes homologous recombination with a second Ty1 element located on another place in the genome. There are data in the literature (Winn 2003) indicating an activation of homologous recombination by elevated ROS levels. Given the importance of having an activation of Ty1 mobility in *rho*⁻ cells only after treatment with H_2O_2, Southern blot experiments were performed to differentiate *de novo* transposition from gene conversion (Figure 2). DNA samples isolated from *rho*⁺ transposants induced with MMS or H_2O_2 have dispersed bands in addition to the 5kb band of the parental insertion. These bands indicated *de novo* transposition events in different locations of the genome. In *rho*⁻ transposants such additional bands were found only after treatment with H_2O_2 and not with MMS. This result evidenced that the supply of ROS by addition of H_2O_2 to the cell culture activates a process of Ty1 transposition *de novo* and not by gene conversion. In addition these results evidence that the overall enhanced level of ROS and not the increased production of a particular oxygen species is involved in the induction of Ty1 mobility by carcinogens.

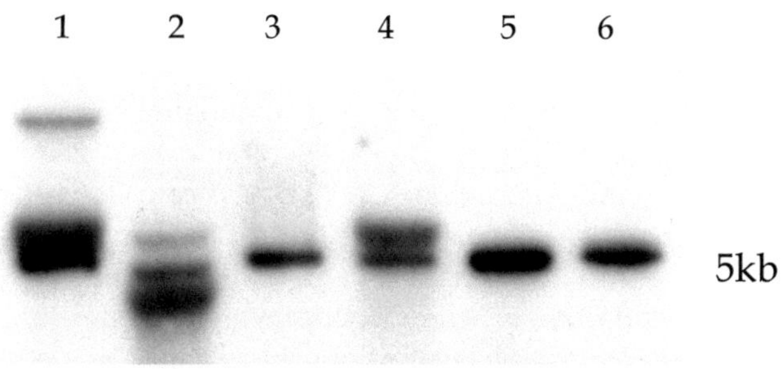

Lanes 1, 2, 3: DNA from *rho*⁺ cells; lanes 4, 5, 6 – DNA from *rho*⁻ cells. Lanes 1 and 4 – cells treated with 1mM H_2O_2 for 30 minutes. Lanes 2 and 5 – cells treated with 3.5mM MMS for 30 minutes. Lanes 3 and 6 – control cells. DNA was digested with *PvuII* and probed with *HIS3*. The 5kb fragment indicates the position of parental TymHis3AI insertion while dispersed bands represent *de novo* transposition events.

Fig. 2. Southern blot analysis of Ty1 retrotransposants

The accumulated data clarify to some extent the molecular mechanism of the selective Ty1 test response to carcinogens. The early work of Wilkie & Evans (1982) suggesting that in yeast cells carcinogens primarily attack the mitochondria, found nowadays its explanation and support in the observation that most, if not all, carcinogenic genotoxins generate high levels of ROS. The generated oxidative stress has different after-effects for the cells, including DNA damages. The oxidative DNA damages act in concert with the DNA damages caused directly by the carcinogens to labilize genome structure, which seems to be one of the first step towards neoplastic differentiation of the cell (Bertram 2001; Garfinkel 2005). Numerous studies (Lesage & Todeschini 2005; Nyswaner et al. 2008; Salmon et al. 2004; Tucker & Fields 2004) indicated the role of DNA damages, induced directly by the carcinogens, in the activation of the Ty1 mobility.

Some of our data, however, suggest an alternative explanation. When *S. cerevisiae* cells are deficient in production of ROS, the treatment with carcinogens does not activate Ty1 mobility, although there are no reasons to suppose that direct DNA damages are not generated by the genotoxin. Cells with compromised production of ROS (*rho*⁻, *sco1*Δ) respond with a dose-dependent increase of Ty1 mobility only if the missing ROS are supplied to the culture. The use of N-acetylcysteine to scavenge the burst of $O_2^{\cdot-}$ following treatment with carcinogens also resulted in lack of activation the Ty1 transposition despite the appearance of direct DNA damages caused by the carcinogen. Opposite results were obtained with menadione, a generator of $O_2^{\cdot-}$ for which literature data (Cojocel et al. 2006) did not support a direct DNA damaging effect. Menadione increased Ty1 transposition without any additional treatment with DNA damaging agent. Finally, cultivation at temperatures at 15-20°C instead of 30°C increases Ty1 transposition (Paquin & Williamson 1986) because of increased ROS production (Zhang et al. 2003) at suboptimal temperatures and not because of the appearance of DNA damages. Together, these data evidence that the increased ROS level may have an independent key role on the induction of Ty1 transposition by carcinogens. We suppose that in cells with functioning mitochondrial oxidative phosphorylation, the carcinogen-induced burst in ROS production is the major initiator of Ty1 transposition. The effect of the direct carcinogen-induced DNA damages is later multiplied by the appearance of secondary oxidative DNA damages due to the already existing oxidative stress. Cells with compromised mitochondrial oxidative phosphorylation can not produce the major initiator in the Ty1 transposition process and the carcinogen activated induction of transposition can not take place in such cells.

Thus, the selective positive answer of Ty1 test to carcinogens is due to activation of Ty1 transposition by the burst of ROS generated by carcinogenic genotoxins. Noncarcinogenic mutagens are not strong ROS generators in *S. cerevisiae* cells and therefore give negative results in the Ty1 test. Both, carcinogens and noncarcinogenic mutagens are DNA damaging agents and the discrimination between the two kinds of genotoxins in Ty1 test is based on the ROS generating capacity of carcinogens which is not an intrinsic property of noncarcinogenic mutagens. These conclusions have been made on the basis of results obtained with 48 carcinogenic and 12 noncarcinogenic but mutagenic genotoxins studied till now in the Ty1 test. Given a number of genotoxins with carcinogenic and/or mutagenic potential of several hundreds, we can well believe that our current interpretation of the molecular mechanism underlying the selective positive response of Ty1 test to carcinogens may undergo some changes depending on the results obtained in future studies.

7. Applicability of Ty1 test: Advantages and shortcomings

7.1 Advantages

The Ty1 test is a short-term test based on fast growing yeast cells and results with this assay are obtained in 5 days. The test is easy to perform and requires expertise at the level of technicians. The usage of only one strain as tester cells makes possible the study of a number of samples per day by one person. The characterization of the test required repetitions to obtain statistically reliable results, but the presence or absence of carcinogenic activities in the studied sample is obvious after the first implementation of the Ty1 test. The accomplishment of the test does not require special equipment and can be performed in every microbiological laboratory. *S. cerevisiae* cells have an intrinsic P_{450}/P_{488} based metabolic system which can be activated by a change in cultivation from low to high dextrose medium. Although the results in Tables are presented with usage of exogenously added S9 mix, very similar values were obtained in almost all experiments using the endogenous metabolic system of the tester 551 cells. The utilization of the intrinsic metabolic activation system in the tester strain further lowers the anyway low cost of the assay.

A significant advantage of the Ty1 test is its ability to respond positively to carcinogens and negatively to noncarcinogenic mutagens. The advantage of having a selective answer to carcinogenic genotoxins becomes evident when the Ty1 test is used at the beginning of a battery of tests in mutagenicity/carcinogenicity studies. Most short-term tests in bacteria or mammalian cells have been designed primarily for hazard identification of genotoxicity and thus represent the starting point in the process of risk assessment. The answer of the important question about the carcinogenic or not carcinogenic nature of a substance is obtained at the end of the battery and is given by studies of the genotoxin in long-term tests. The implementation of Ty1 assay at the beginning of the study will give in 5 days the information about presence or absence of carcinogenic potential of the genotoxin and will spare time, efforts and costs. Therefore, the Ty1 assays is an indicator test that provides evidence of carcinogenicity and is thus an indicator of carcinogenic potential.

Another important advantage of Ty1 test is its wide range in detection of carcinogens. Several carcinogenic genotoxins not detectable by the other short-term tests were tested and found to give positive results in Ty1 assay. The following reasons can be considered in explanation the wider range of Ty1 test in carcinogen detection.

First, the tester cells have mutationally increased cellular permeability to genotoxins which facilitates the uptake of carcinogens in otherwise low permeable, and therefore low sensitive *S. cerevisiae* cells. Second, the Ty1 test is based on activation the transposition of a Ty1 transposon which is a typical genetic retroelement with structure, function and cell-cycle analogous to the known oncogenic retroviruses. Similarities in regulation of certain steps of Ty1 transposition and neoplastic differentiation of cells were detected, which might explain to some extent the selective character of Ty1 test response to wider range of carcinogens. Finally and probably most importantly, the molecular mechanism of the positive Ty1 test response is principally different compared to other assays. Most short-term tests were constructed to detect one genetic *end-point* raised by one, or several (but not all) carcinogens. On the opposite, the positive response of Ty1 test is due to induction the *initiation step* of the transposition process. Instead of detecting a DNA-damage as end-product of the effect of some carcinogens, the Ty1 test is based on activation the start of a process. This activation is due to increased ROS levels generated by the carcinogens, which seems to be a property common to most, if not all, carcinogens. We consider such molecular mechanism of carcinogen detection as important in explanation the selective Ty1 test response to wider range of carcinogens.

7.2 Shortcomings

The advantage of Ty1 test to selectively detect carcinogens may be assessed as a shortcoming, if the test is used alone in environmental studies. Results obtained with laboratory genotoxins and in field studies evidenced a negative response of the test to noncarcinogenic mutagens. Thus, environmental samples taken from regions polluted with mutagens that are not carcinogenic will remain silent in the test. A way to overcome this shortcoming is to use the Ty1 assay for environmental studies together with a short-term test detecting mutations, if information about the general pollution of the region is required.

Another disadvantage of Ty1 test would be that the assay will give positive results with substances that are ROS generators in *S. cerevisiae*, irrespective of their carcinogenic or noncarcinogenic nature. The ROS generators represent a small group of chemicals used for research only and not found as environmental pollutants. Their carcinogenic potential is not well known and remains to be studied in the future.

A positive result of environmental sample in the Ty1 test means that the region this sample was collected from is polluted with carcinogen(s). The test does not show if one or a mixture of carcinogens are present in the sample. This feature of the Ty1 test is shared by the other short-term tests, as well.

The Ty1 test is a quantitative assay in the sense that every transposition event of the marked Ty1 element activated by the studied genotoxin gives rise to one His^+ colony. A concentration dependence of the positive answer was found for all studied carcinogens in the test, suggesting that higher fold increase of Ty1 transposition means higher concentration of the genotoxin in the sample. However, the activation of the Ty1 transposition process depends on increased ROS generated by the genotoxins. Studies, now in progress, indicate that different carcinogens produce various levels of ROS in *S. cerevisiae* and that the fold increase of Ty1 transposition depends on ROS level and not on the concentration of the genotoxins. Therefore, the fold increase of transposition reflects the ROS generating capacity of carcinogen(s) and not the amount of the genotoxin in the studied sample. The property of Ty1 test to give a quantitative measure of carcinogen's effect has to be taken into consideration only when different concentrations of one particular genotoxin are studied.

7.3 Fields of applications

The Ty1 test can be successfully used in research to study carcinogenicity of chemicals, including such applied in agriculture, nutrition and pharmacy. A positive answer of the test would be a strong indicator for carcinogenic potential of the studied substance or drug. The test can also be applied to study ROS generators and scavengers. Since the increase of Ty1 transposition depends on the ROS level, a decrease in the rate of transposition caused by an added substance indicates scavenging properties of this substance.

Another application of the Ty1 test is its usage in control studies of food products. Some foods, such as smoked meat, fish, cheese, etc., have to be checked according to the requirements of the European Commission for Nutrition, for presence of carcinogens that accumulate on the surface during product's processing. The usage of liquid additives instead of wooden smoke does not guarantee a full absence of carcinogens in food products.

The usage of Ty1 test in environmental studies has been described in order to better characterize the assay. In this research environmental samples were studied in Ty1 test and chemically analyzed for presence of genotoxins. The results obtained showed a positive response of Ty1 test to samples from regions polluted with carcinogens in amounts exceeding the accepted ecological standards and negative results with samples from region not polluted with carcinogens. The high sensitivity of the test, its selectivity towards carcinogenic pollutants and the absence of false positive responses substantiated the inclusion of Ty1 assay in the battery of tests used by the National Executive Environmental Agency (Sofia, Bulgaria) to control pollution of environment.

8. Acknowledgements

We thank Dr A. Tzagoloff (New York, USA), Dr W. Scott-Moye-Rowley (Iowa, USA) and Dr. R. Akada (Tokiwadai, Japan) for the plasmids. This study was supported partly by the Science for Peace program of NATO, Grant №977977 given to P.V.

9. References

Bajpayee M, Pandey AK, Parmar D, Dhawan A (2005) Current status of short-term tests for evaluation of genotoxicity, mutagenicity and carcinogenicity of environmental chemicals and NCEs. *Toxicology Mechanisms and Methods* 15:155-180.

Barros MH, Bandy B, Tahara EB, Kowaltowski AJ (2004) Higher respiratory activity decreases mitochondrial reactive oxygen release and increases life span in *Saccharomyces cerevisiae. J Biol Chem* 279(48):49883-8.

Bernstein H, Bernstein C, Payne CM, Dvorakova K, Garewal H (2005) Bile acids as carcinogens in human gastrointestinal cancers. *Mutat Res* 589(1):47-65.

Bertram JS (2001) The molecular genetics of carcinogenesis. Mol Aspect Med. 21: 167-223.

Bradshaw VA, McEntee K (1989) DNA damage activates transcription and transposition of yeast Ty retrotransposons. *Mol Gen Genet* 218(3):465-74.

Brennan RJ, Schiestl RH (1998) Free radicals generated in yeast by the *Salmonella* test-negative carcinogens benzene, thiourea and auramine. Mutat Res 403:65-73.

Cannon RE, Spalding JW, Trampus CS, Szezesniak CJ, Virgil K, Humble MC, Tennan RW (1997) Kinetics of wound induced v-Ha-ras transgene expression and papilloma development in transgenic Tg.AC mice. *Mol Carcinogen* 20:108-114.

Carls N, Schiestl RH (1994) Evaluation of the yeast DEL assay with 10 compounds selected by the International Program on Chemical Safety for the evaluation of short-term tests for carcinogens. *Mutat Res* 320 :293-303.

Clive DK, Johnson D, Spectre JE, Batson AG, Brown MMM (1979) Validation and characterization of the L1578Y TK+/- mouse lymphoma assay system. *Mutat Res* 59:61-108.

Cojocel C, Novotny L, Vachalkova (2006) Mutagenic and carcinogenic potential of menadione. *Neoplasma* 53:316-323.

Curcio MJ and Garfinkel DJ (1991) Single-step selection for Ty1 element retrotransposition. *Proc Natl Acad Sci* 88:936–940.

Curcio MJ, Kenny AE, Moore S, Garfinkel DJ, Weintraub M, Gamache ER, Scholes DT (2007) S-phase checkpoint pathways stimulate the mobility of the retrovirus-like transposon Ty1. *Mol Cell Biol* 27(24): 8874-85.

De Nobel JG, Barnett JA (1991) Passage of molecules through yeast cell walls: a brief essay-review. *Yeast*7(4):313-23.

Dimitrov M, Venkov P, Pesheva M (2010) The positive response of Ty1 retrotransposition test to carcinogens is due to increased levels of reactive oxygen species generated by the genotoxins. *Arch Toxicol* 85:67-74.

Donkin SG, Ohlson DL, Teaf CM (2000) Properties of metals. In: Williams PL, James RC, Roberts (Eds) Principles of Toxicology: Environmental and industrial applications, 2nd edn. John Wiley and Sons Inc., pp325-345.

Dujon, B (1981) Mitochondrial genes, mutants, maps - a review, In: Schweyen RJ, Wolf K, Kandewitz (Eds.) *Mitochondria, Walter de Gryuter*, Berlin, pp1-24.

Eastmond DA, Macgregor JT, Slesinski RS (2008) Trivalent chromium: assessing the genotoxic risk of an essential trace element and widely used human and animal nutritional supplement. *Crit Rev Toxicol* 38(3):173-90.

Epstein CB, Waddle JA, Hale W, Davé V, Thornton J, Macatee TL, Garner HR, Butow RA (2001) Genome-wide responses to mitochondrial dysfunction. *Mol Biol Cell* 12:297-308.

Eastmond DA, Hartwig A, Anderson D, Anwar WA, Cimono MC, Dobrev I, Douglas GR, Nohmi T, Phollips DH, Vickers C (2009) Mutagenicity testing for chemical risk assessment: update of the WHO/IPCS harmonized scheme. Mutagenesis 24:341-349.

Fridovich I (1997) Superoxide anion radical ($O_2^{-\cdot}$), superoxide dismutases, and related matters. *J Biol Chem* 272(30):18515-7.

Galloway SM (2000) Cytotoxicity and chromosomal aberrations *in vitro*: Experience in industry and the case for an upper limit on toxicity in the aberration assay. *Environ Mol Mutagen* 35:191-201.

Garfinkel DJ (2005) Genome evolution mediated by Ty elements in *Saccharomyces. Cytogenet Genome Res* 110(1-4):63-9.

Garfinkel DJ, Stefanisko KM, Nyswaner KM, Moore SP, Oh J, Hughes SH (2006) Retrotransposon suicide: formation of Ty1 circles and autointegration via a central DNA flap. J Virology 80:11920-934.

Glerum DM, Shtanko A, Tzagoloff A (1996) *SCO1* and *SCO2* act as high copy suppressors of a mitochondrial copper recruitment defect in *Saccharomyces cerevisiae. J Biol Chem* 271:20531-5.

Goldman R, Enewold L, Pellizzari E, Beach JB, Bowman ED, Krishnan SS, Shields PG (2001) Smoking increases carcinogenic polycyclic aromatic hydrocarbons in human lung tissue. *Cancer Res.* 61(17):6367-71.

Herrero E, Ros J, Bellí G, Cabiscol E (2008) Redox control and oxidative stress in yeast cells. *Biochimica et Biophysica Acta* 1780:1217–1235.

Hu H (2002) Human health and heavy metal exposure, In: McCarth M (Ed) Life Support: The environment and human health. *MIT Press*, Ch. 4.

Ito H, Fukuda Y, Murata K, and Kimura A (1983) Transformation of intact yeast cells treated with alkali cations. *J Bacteriol* 153:163–168.

Ito N, Imada K, Hirose K, Shirai T (1998) Medium term bioassay for carcinogenicity of chemical mixture. *Environ Health Perspect* 106:1331-1336.

Jamieson DJ (1992) *Saccharomyces cerevisiae* has distinct adaptive responses to both hydrogen peroxide and menadione. *J Bacteriol* 174(20):6678-81.

Jerónimo C, Nomoto S, Caballero OL, Usadel H, Henrique R, Varzim G, Oliveira J, Lopes C, Fliss MS and Sidransky D (2001) Mitochondrial mutations in early stage prostate cancer and bodily fluids. *Oncogene* 20(37):5195-8.

Johnson KL, Tucker JD, Nath J (1998) Frequency, distribution and clonality of chromosome damage in human lymphocytes by multi-colour FISH. *Mutagenesis* 13:217-227.

Kajiwara Y, Ajimi S, Hosokawa A, Mackawa K (1997) Improvement of carcinogen detection in the BALB/3T3 cell transformation assay by using a rich basal medium supplemented with low concentration of serum and some growth factors. *Mutat Res* 393:81-90.

Kepes F, Schekman R. (1988) The yeast *SEC53* gene encodes phosphomannomutase. *J Biol Chem* 263(19):9155-61.

Kirchner J, Connolly CM, Sandmayer SB (1995) Requirement of RNA polymerase III transcription factors for *in vitro* position-specific integration of a retroviruslike element. *Science* 267:1488-1491.

LeBeouf RA, Kerkaert KA, Aardema MJ, Isfort RJ (1999) Use of Syrian hamster embryo and BALB/c3T3 cell transformation for assessing the carcinogenic potential of chemicals, *IARC Sci Publ* 146:409-425.

Lesage P, Todeschini AL (2005) Happy together: the life and times of Ty retrotransposons and their hosts. *Cytogenet Genome Res* 110(1-4):70-90.

Levina A, Lay PA (2008) Chemical properties and toxicity of chromium(III) nutritional supplements. *Chem Res Toxicol* 21(3):563-71.

Li AP, Corver JH, Choy WN, Hsie AW, Gupta RS, Loveday KS, O'Neil JP, Riddle JP, Stankowski Jr.LF, Yang II (1987) A guide for the performance of the Chinese hamster ovary cells/hypoxanthine guanine phosphoryl transferse gene mutation assay. *Mutat Res* 189:135-141.

Lin SJ, Kaeberlein M, Andalis AA, Sturtz LA, Defossez PA, Culotta VC, Fink GR and Guarente L (2002) Calorie restriction extends *Saccharomyces cerevisiae* lifespan by increasing respiration. *Nature* 418:344-8.

Llorens C, Muñoz-Pomer A, Bernad L, Botella H, Moya A (2009) Network dynamics of eukaryotic LTR retroelements beyond phylogenetic trees. *Biol Direct.* 4:41.

Mewes HW, Albermann K, Bähr M, Frishman D, Gleissner A, Hani J, Heumann K, Kleine K, Maierl A, Oliver SG, Pfeiffer F, Zollner A (1997) Overview of the yeast genome. *Nature* 387(6634):737.

Morita T, Iwamoto Y, Shimizu T, Masuzawa T, Yanagihara Y (1989) Mutagenicity tests with a permeable mutant of yeast on carcinogens showing false-negative in *Salmonella* assay. *Chem Pharm Bull* 37(2):407-9.

Neri M, Fucic A, Knudsen LE, Lando C, Merlo F, Bonassi S (2003) Micronuclei frequency in children exposed to environmental mutagens: A review. *Mutat Res* 544:243-298.

Nguyên DT, Alarco AM, Raymond M (2001) Multiple Yap1p-binding sites mediate induction of the yeast major facilitator FLR1 gene in response to drugs, oxidants, and alkylating agents. *J Biol Chem* 276:1138-45.

Nyswaner KM, Checkley MA, Yi M, Stephens RM and Garfinkel DJ (2008) Chromatin-associated genes protect the yeast genome from Ty1 insertional mutagenesis. *Genetics* 178:197-214.

Paquin CE and Williamson VM (1984) Temperature effects on the rate of Ty transposition. *Science* 226:53-55.

Parry EM, Parry JM, Corso C, Doherty A, Haddad F, Hermine TF, Johnson G, Kayani M, Quick E, Warr T, Williamson J (2002) Detection and characterization of mechanisms of action of aneugenic chemicals. *Mutagenesis* 17:509-521.

Parry JM, Davies PJ, Evans WE (1976) The effects of "cell age" upon the lethal effects of chemical and physical mutagens in the yeast, *Saccharomyces cerevisiae. Mol Gen Genet* 146:27-35.

Pesheva M, Krastanova O, Staleva L, Deutcheva V, Hadzhitodorov M, Venkov P (2005) The Ty1 transposition assay: a new short - term test for detection of carcinogens. *J Microb Meth* 61:1-8.

Ramel C, Cederberg H, Magnusson J, Vogel E, Natarajan AT, Mullender LH, Nivard JM, Parry JM, Leyson A, Comendador MA, Sierra LM, Ferreiro JA, Consuegra S (1996) Somatic recombination, gene amplification and cancer. *Mutat Res* 353(1-2):85-107.

Ribeiro-dos-Santos G, Schenberg AC, Gardner DC, Oliver SG (1997) Enhancement of Ty transposition at the ADH4 and ADH2 loci in meiotic yeast cells. *Mol Gen Genet* 254:555-561.

Rodriguez-Reyes R, Morales-Rmirez (2003) Sister chromatide exchange induction and the course of DNA duplication, two mechanisms of sister chromatide exchange induction by ENU and the role of BrdU. *Mutagenesis* 18:65-72.

Roeder GS, Fink GR (1982) Movement of yeast transposable elements by gene conversion. *Proc Natl Acad Sci U S A* 79(18):5621-5.

Rolfe M, Banks G (1986) Induction of yeast Ty element transcription by ultraviolet light. *Nature* 319:339-340.

Salamone MF (1981) Toxicity of 41 carcinogens and noncarcinogenic analogs. *Prog Mutat Res* 1:682-688.

Salmon TB, Evert BA, Song B, Doetsch PW (2004) Biological consequences of oxidative stress-induced DNA damage in *Saccharomyces cerevisiae. Nucleic Acids Res* 32(12):3712-23.

Scandalios JG (2005) Oxidative stress: molecular perception and transduction of signals triggering antioxidant gene defenses. *Braz J Med Biol Res* 38:995-1014.

Schumacher AJ, Hache G, MaeDuff DA, Brown WL, Harris RS (2008) The DNA deaminase activity of human APOBEC3G is required for Ty1, MusD and human immunodeficiency virus type 1 restriction. *J Virol* 82: 2652-2660.

Scott D, Galloway SM, Marshal RR, Ishidate M, Brusick D, Ashby J, Myhr BC (1991) Genotoxicity under extreme culture conditions. A report from ICPEMC task group 9. *Mutat Res* 257(2):147-205.

Sherman F, Fink GR, Hicks GB (2001) Methods in Yeast Genetics: A Laboratory Manual. *Cold Spring Harbor Laboratory Press, Plainview, NY.*

Singh NP, Tice RR, Stephens RE, Schneider EI (1991) A microgel electrophoresis technique for the direct quantification of DNA damage and repair in individual fibroblasts cultured on microscope slides. *Mutat Res* 252:289-296.

Split G, Hartmann A (2005) The comet assay: a sensitive genotoxicity test for the detection of DNA damages. *Meth Mol Biol* 291: 85-95.

Staleva L (1998) A principally new test for detection of mutagens and carcinogens. PhD thesis, Institute of Molecular Biology, *Bulg Acad Sciences*.

Staleva L, Waltscheva L, Golovinsky E, Venkov P (1996) Enhanced cell permeability increases the sensitivity of a yeast test for mutagens. *Mutat Res* 370(2):81-9.

Staleva LS and Venkov PV (2001) Activation of Ty transposition by mutagens. *Mutat Res* 474:93–103.

Stamenova R, Dimitrov M, Stoycheva T, Pesheva M, Venkov P, Tsvetkov Ts (2008) Transposition of *Saccharomyces cerevisiae* Ty1 retrotransposon is activated by improper cryopreservation. *Cryobiology* 56:241-247.

Stoner GD, Shimkin MB (1982) StrainA mouse lung bioassay. *J Amer Coll Toxicol* 1:145-169.

Stoycheva T, Massardo DR, Pesheva M, Venkov P, Volf K, Giudice L, Pontieri P (2007) Ty1 transposition induced by carcinogens in *Saccharomyces cerevisiae* yeast depends on mitochondrial function. *Gene* 389:212-218.

Stoycheva T, Pesheva M, Venkov P (2010) The role of reactive oxygen species in the induction of Ty1 retrotransposition in *Saccharomyces cerevisiae*. *Yeast* 27:259-267.

Stoycheva T, Pesheva M, Venkov P (2005) Transposition of *Saccharomyces cerevisiae* Ty1 retrotransposon depends on the function of mitochondria. *Biotechnol Biotechol Eq* 19(2):116-121.

Stoycheva T, Venkov P, Tsvetkov Ts (2007) Mutagenic effect of freezing on mitochondrial DNA of *Saccharomyces cerevisiae*. *Cryobiology* 54:243–250.

Szeles A (2002) Fluorescence *in situ* hybridization (FISH) in the molecular cytogenesis of cancer. *Acta Microbiol Immunol Hung* 49:64-80.

Temple MD, Perrone GG, Dawes IW, (2005) Complex cellular responses to reactive oxygen species. *Trends Cell Biol* 15:319–326.

Tennant RW, French JE, Spalding Jr (1995) Identification of chemical carcinogens and assessing potential risk in short-term bioassays using transgenic mouse models. *Environ Health Perspect* 103:942-950.

Toyoyka T, Ibuki Y (2007) DNA damage induced by coexposure to PAHs and light. Envir *Tox Pharm* 23:256-273.

Tucker CL, Fields S (2004) Quantitative genome-wide analysis of yeast deletion strain sensitivities to oxidative and chemical stress. Comp Funct Genomics 5(3):216-24.

Verschueren E (2001) *Handbook of Environmental Data on Organic Chemicals*, 4th edn, Vol.1. Wiley, New York.

Wegrzyn G, Czyz A (2003) Detection of mutagenic pollution of natural environment using microbiological assays, *J Appl Microbiol* 95:1175-1181

Wilkie D, Evans I (1982) Mitochondria and the yeast cells surface: implications of carcinogenesis. *TIBS* 76:147-151.

Winn LM (2003) Homologous recombination initiated by benzene metabolites: a potential role of oxidative stress. *Toxicol Sci* 72:143-149.

YARC (1990) Monographs of the evaluation of carcinogenic risks to humans. Vol 49, YARC Scientific Publications, YSRC, Lyon.

Zhang L, Onda K, Imai R, Fukuda R, Horiuchi H, Ohta A. (2003) Growth temperature downshift induces antioxidant response in *Saccharomyces cerevisiae. Biochem Biophys Res Commun* 307:308-14.

Zimmermann FK, Kern R, Rasenberger H (1975) A yeast strain for simultaneous detection of induced mitotic crossingover, mitotic gene conversion and reverse mutation. *Mutat Res* 28:381-388.

Zlotnik KH, Femande MP, Bowers B, Cabib E (1989) Mannoproteins form an external cell wall layer determines wall porosity in *Saccharomyces cerevisiae. J Bacteriol* 195:1018–1026.

6

Isolation and Detection of Carcinogenic Nucleic Acid Adducts

Dickson M. Wambua[1], Amanda L. Brownstone[1], Charles A. Barnes[3] and Norman H. L. Chiu[1,2,*]

[1]Department of Chemistry & Biochemistry, University of North Carolina at Greensboro, Greensboro, NC,
[2]Department of Nanoscience, Joint School of Nanoscience and Nanoengineering, University of North Carolina at Greensboro, NC,
[3]Department of Chemistry, Iowa State University, Ames, IA, USA

1. Introduction

In general, nucleic acid adducts are formed when harmful chemical compounds react covalently with cellular DNA or RNA molecules. With only four natural nucleobases in DNA or RNA, identical nucleic acid adducts can theoretically occur at multiple positions within the human genome or transcriptome. The frequency of nucleic acid adduction is further increased by the reactivity of DNA or RNA to form adducts with many different types of chemicals, which include both exogenous compounds that our bodies have been exposed and endogenous compounds that are generated through normal metabolic activities in our bodies.[1,2] Some exogenous compounds may require metabolic activation prior to the formation of nucleic acid adducts, whereas others may react directly with nucleic acids. If DNA adducts are not effectively removed by the DNA repair mechanism, the adducts can directly interfere with DNA replication and transcription.[3] Similarly, the presence of adducts in RNA molecules can affect their biological functions. From the results of many experimental studies, the association of either DNA adducts or RNA adducts to cancer have already been well established. In the case of DNA adducts, it is widely recognized as the key element for the onset of carcinogenesis. Both DNA adducts and RNA adducts are, therefore, important biomarkers for cancer research, which include the monitoring of exposure to carcinogens, genetic mutation, DNA repair and so on. Similar to the analysis of other cancer biomarkers, both identification and quantification of nucleic acid adducts are required. Prior to the detection of nucleic acid adducts, it is important to ensure the biological or clinical samples are collected and stored properly. Equally important, the isolation of genomic DNA or RNA has to be carried out with high efficiency, which includes the yield and purity of selected material, reproducibility and the rate of sample throughput. For the detection of nucleic acid adducts, the requirements can be divided into the following order:

---

* Corresponding Author

1. *Limit of Detection*. First and foremost is the ability to detect the presence of the adduct of interest. The detection signal that corresponds to a specific adduct should be at least two times above the background noise which originates from either the sample matrix or electronic components in an analytical instrumentation.
2. *Selectivity*. The major analytical challenge for the analysis of nucleic acid adducts is that the ratio between unmodified nucleotides and adducts can be as high as 10^{12} : 1. To achieve an accurate measurement, it is very important to be able to select or separate the adduct of interest from other nucleotides that have not been modified.
3. *Specificity*. For the analysis of nucleic acid adducts, specificity refers to the ability to distinguish the target adduct from the other possible adducts, including different isomers, that may co-exist in the same sample. In the case of mass spectrometric methods, this can be easily achieved by using a mass spectrometer that can provide high mass resolution (e.g. Orbitrap from Thermo Scientific).
4. *Quantitation*. As mentioned above, it is important to be able to accurately determine the amount of target adduct in a biological sample. To achieve absolute quantitation, the construction of a calibration graph with the dilutions of a pure standard is required. This can be a challenge simply because many pure standards of nucleic acid adducts are not available.
5. *Reproducibility*. It is important to ensure the method being used to measure a target adduct is reproducible which includes both intraday and interday reproducibility.
6. *Sample Throughput*. With a wide variety of nucleic acid adducts and their high frequency of occurrence in a genome and transcriptome, the number of assays that are required in a specific study, especially in a clinical related study, can be relatively high. Thus, it is necessary to consider the time which is required to complete every step in the method being used as well as how many samples can be processed in parallel at the same time.
7. *Cost*. For measuring a relatively high number of samples, the cost of running a particular method for each sample can add up to a prohibitive level. In general, the higher the sensitivity of the method, the less sample and reagent are required. Also, the smaller the number of experimental steps is involved in a selected method, the fewer reagents are required.

To address these challenges for analyzing nucleic acid adducts, a number of different methods have been designed and developed.[4,5,6,7,8,9] Among those methods, LC-MS is the most commonly used analytical technique for carrying out the end point measurements of nucleic acid adducts. However, different samples or different adducts often pose their unique challenges. In other words, there is no single analytical technique that can be considered as a universal technique for detecting nucleic acid adducts. Unlike some of the recent publications, in which only the use of one specific analytical technique was discussed, this chapter provides an overview of the entire process for analyzing nucleic acid adducts. This chapter begins with a section on the introduction and challenges of nucleic acid adduct analysis. In the second section, the isolation and initial characterization of genomic DNA or specific groups of cellular RNA are discussed. Various analytical methods that have been developed for the detection of nucleic acid adducts are discussed in the third and fourth section, which also includes the rationale for selecting each detection method. It is, however, not our intention to review the analysis of each specific nucleic acid adduct that have been reported in the literature.

2. Methods

2.1 Isolation of genomic DNA and specific groups of cellular RNA

With the advance in the techniques for isolating nucleic acids from cellular samples, the analysis of nucleic acids has become an indispensable tool for studying the biological processes in different types of living organisms. As shown in Figure 1, sample preparation is the most important step preceding any specific type of nucleic acid measurement. For instance, the purpose of proper sampling is to ensure that a representative sample is collected, whose identity and composition is representative of the true *in-situ* abundance. Equally important, the integrity of DNA and RNA should be preserved to ensure trustworthiness and relevance of the data would be obtained in the downstream measurements. This section will cover the current methods for isolating cellular DNA or RNA with high yields and purity as well as the best practice on storing the samples.

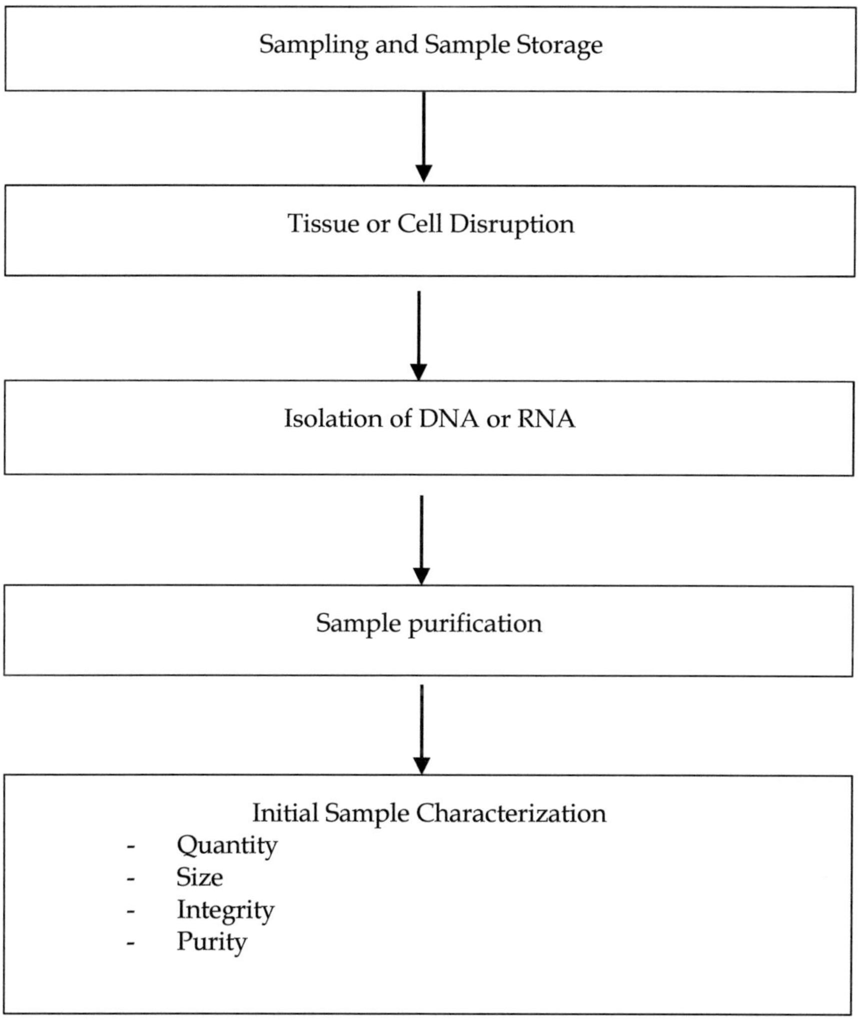

Fig. 1. Schematic diagram of work flow for preparing nucleic acid adduct samples

In general, the isolation of nucleic acids is dependent on the efficiency on disrupting the tissues or cells, the inactivation of nucleases such as deoxyribonuclease (DNase) or ribonuclease (RNase), and the removal of any proteins that may be structurally associated with nucleic acids. Since the quality of any downstream process including the nucleic acid measurements is dependent on the purity of isolated nucleic acids, great care should be taken to avoid any contamination. The most common contaminants include cellular proteins, carbohydrates, lipids, or the presence of RNA in isolated DNA and vice versa.[10] An extensive review on the effects of nucleic acid sample preparations on downstream applications was recently published by GE Healthcare.[11]

The procedures used for sample preparation prior to the isolation of cellular nucleic acids are critical for success. Special care should be taken to prevent sample degradation by nucleases during and after isolation. For example, the degradation of a DNA or RNA biomolecules may hinder a downstream measurement where the nucleic acid is required to bind to a complementary probe such as in microarray analysis. Some indicators of nucleic acid degradation or contamination may include extra products in PCR reactions, failure or reduced success in steps involving nucleic acid modification or restriction using enzymes. A classic signature of nuclease contamination in DNA samples is the characteristic ladder like separation or smear when the DNA is electrophoresed in an agarose gel. In some circumstances, it is necessary to isolate both genomic DNA and RNA from the same sample and this is discussed later in the chapter.[12]

Many commercial kits for the isolation of nucleic acids have been developed but the challenges of sample preparation still remain. These challenges include the availability of very small sample sizes, the ability to eliminate all contaminating materials that may interfere with downstream measurements and the fact that degradation of nucleic acids starts immediately after sample collection. In some cases, samples are difficult to disrupt so as to get to the nucleic acids. It is also challenging to isolate both DNA and RNA from the same sample, to isolate small RNA that are less than 200 nucleotides long, to detect nucleic acids arising from viruses in collected samples, or to detect RNA transcripts which are expressed in low abundance.[13]

2.2 Sampling and sample storage

Prior to the isolation of nucleic acids, it is important to determine which is the nucleic acid of interest (i.e. DNA or RNA), the type of sample that will be collected, and an estimate of how much nucleic acid materials will be required. The limit of detection of the technique to be used for downstream measurements, and its tolerance to contamination should also be considered. All these information are needed for choosing the most suitable isolation method.14 Nucleic acids have been successfully isolated from tissue, cell culture, bacteria, yeast, fungi, virus, soil, fecal samples, and biofluids such as blood, serum, plasma, lymph, cerebral spinal fluid, ascites, saliva, urine, and amniotic fluid. Following the collection of samples, the general guideline is to begin the process of nucleic acid isolation as quickly as possible. In this way, the possible degradation of nucleic acids will be kept to the minimum. If immediate isolation is not possible, the tissue or cellular samples can be mixed with a stabilizing agent (e.g. RNAlater® from Qiagen) or flash frozen the samples in liquid nitrogen and stored at -80°C. In cases where nucleic acids have to be stored at room temperature for extended periods of time, commercial products such as the FTA Cards technology developed by Whatman can be used. In brief, the FTA cards contain chemically conditioned cellulose fiber matrices whose composition quickly lyse the cells, inactivate proteins and immobilize the nucleic acids thereby protecting the samples from degeneration. Once the samples have been spotted on the cards, the cards have to be thoroughly dried and can be stored at room temperature for long term archiving. For the FTA cards, the cellular debris is washed away and the nucleic acids remain bound to the card. Whereas, for the FTA Elute, nucleic acids are eluted from the cards using water at 95°C while contaminants remain bound on the cellulose matrix.[15] Isolated DNA samples are best stored at -20°C in 1X TE buffer. If long term storage is required, the isolated nucleic acids should be dissolved in 70% ethanol and stored at -80°C. Prior to storing the samples, the stock solution should be divided into small aliquots which can avoid the degradation of the sample during the freeze and thaw cycles of the stock solution. It is important to make sure that the buffer used to store the nucleic acids is compatible with the downstream experiments such as PCR, mass spectrometry etc.[16]

2.3 Sample disruption and deactivation of nucleases

DNA is found within the nucleus of the cell, tightly coil around histone proteins and together forming the chromatin, while RNA is present both inside and outside the nucleus. The cell membrane forms a protective and selectively permeable layer around the cellular contents, protecting them from the extracellular environment. In order to isolate nucleic acids from collected samples, the DNA or RNA has to be liberated from the cells first by breaking down the cell membrane and forms a cell lysate, a process known as sample disruption. Cultured cells can be lysed directly. Whereas, solid samples such as tissue sections have to be physically disrupted. Sample disruption should be carried out in such a manner that the integrity of nucleic acids is preserved. A high degree of cell membrane disruption is desired in order to maximize the yield of isolated nucleic acids and prevent problems in subsequent steps such as clogging of purification columns. After sample disruption and homogenization, there should be no visible particulates unless the sample contained non cellular components such as bones or connective tissue. The cell membranes can be disrupted and homogenized in a variety of ways. These disruption methods are classified as either mechanical or non-mechanical.[17]

2.3.1 Mechanical methods of cell disruption

Mechanical cell lysis methods involve breaking the samples by shearing force under liquid nitrogen. The samples are mechanically ground using equipment such as a French press, sonicator, bead mill or homogenizer.[18] Mechanical disruption methods can lead to complete cell disruption but can also cause heating or foaming of the sample. Mechanical methods are used for samples such as animal tissues that require great force to disrupt.[19]

2.3.2 Non-mechanical methods of cell disruption

Non-mechanical methods involve physical, chemical or enzymatic processes. These methods can be used for samples such as cultured cells that do not require strong disruption methods. Physical ways of disrupting samples include decompression, freeze thaw, osmotic shock lysis, desiccation, or thermolysis. For example, the freeze thaw technique uses repeated freezing and thawing of cells to form sharp ice crystals within the cells to disrupt the sample.[20] Osmotic shock lysis technique is dependent on the changes of hydrostatic pressure created by a change in concentration of solutes between a semipermeable cell membrane. The osmotic gradient forces water to flow through the cell membrane, and result in breaking the cells apart. Chemical methods use detergents, salts, solvents, or chelating agents to disrupt the cells. For chemical disruption, chaotropic salts such as guanidinium isothiocyanate disrupt cells by providing a less hydrophobic condition in the sample that in return weakens the hydrophobic interactions within the cell membrane, thus breaking the cell membrane apart. Chaotropic salts also possess the ability to denature nucleases and proteins. Detergent chemical based disruption works by disturbing the hydrophobic interactions of phospholipids that are part of the cell membranes. Enzymatic methods utilize lysozymes and proteases to break down the cell membranes and are mainly used to disrupt cell cultures. Enzymatic treatment is typically followed by sonication, and homogenization by overtaxing in a lysing buffer.21

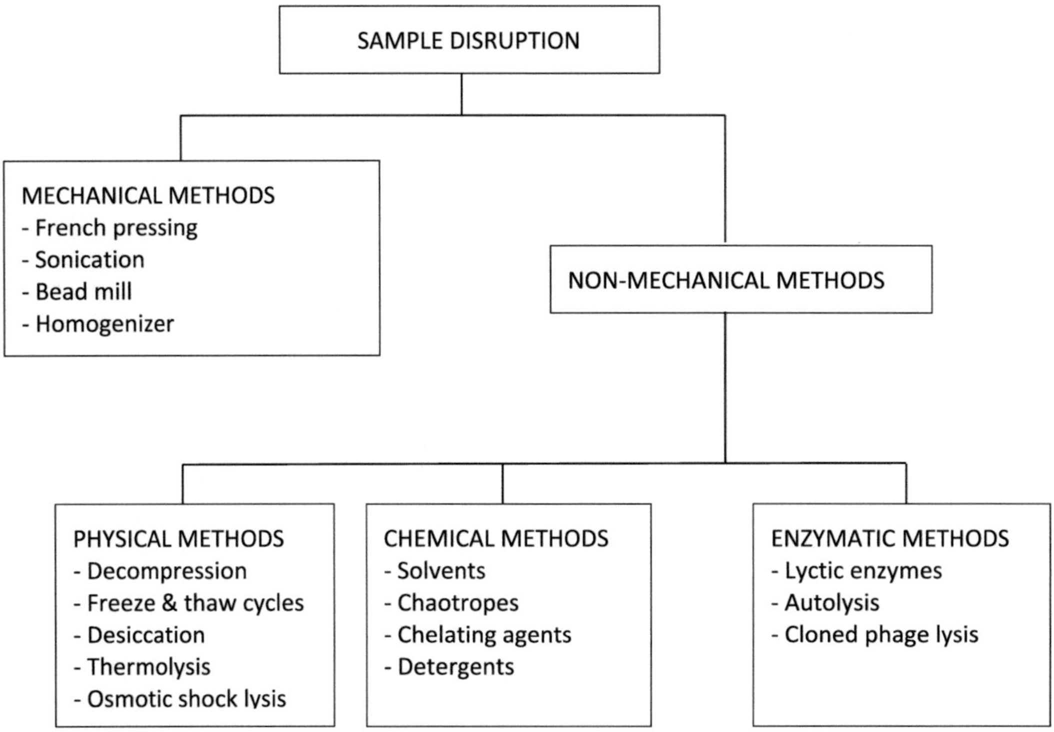

Fig. 2. Summary of sample disruption methods.

Pathological samples are often formalin-fixed and paraffin embedded (FFPE). If FFPE samples have to be used for the isolation of nucleic acids, proper deparafinization using an organic solvent like xylene should be done first.22 As a general rule, it is advisable to use the mildest disruption method possible to avoid mechanical breakdown of nucleic acids, perform the isolation within the shortest period of time by using pre-chilled equipment and use nuclease inhibitors. The choice of purification method will depend on the desired quality and purity of nucleic acids as well as the yield required for downstream analysis.

Disruption of frozen samples is best done in liquid nitrogen rather than letting the samples thaw for the same reasons of limiting nuclease activity.[23]

Usually one of the most important steps towards achieving high quality of nucleic acids is the inactivation of nucleases immediately after the sample is disrupted. Naturally occurring nucleases in the sample can degrade nucleic acids and therefore, during lysis, it is advisable to add a nuclease inhibitor into the lysing buffer. After sample collection, the samples can be flash-frozen using liquid nitrogen or homogenized in the presence of nuclease inactivation solution. Placing sample in a lysing buffer such as guanidinium isothiocyanate can inactivate nucleases. Chelating agents such as EDTA that sequester Mg^{2+} ions which are required for nuclease activity can also be used to prevent nucleic acid degradation by nucleases during storage. Treatment of the sample using proteinase K digests and degrades all proteins, including nucleases. The breakdown of proteins reduces the viscosity of samples and helps in subsequent steps such as filtration.[24] Moreover, nucleases are ubiquitous and can be found in glassware as well as on our fingers. Thus, care should also be taken to avoid contaminating the samples with exogenous nucleases. The use of a clean nuclease-free working area and wearing gloves should always be part of the experimental procedure. Likewise, glassware should be sterilized at 250 °C for two hours.[25]

2.4 DNA isolation techniques

Since the first DNA isolation by the Swiss physician Friedrich Miescher in 1869, numerous protocols have been developed. DNA isolation begins with cell membrane disruption, removal of histone proteins, cell membrane debris and other biomolecules like RNA, lipids and proteins. The common DNA isolation methods are either solution based isolation, silica based methods or anion exchange. Solution based isolation methods use organic solvents such as phenol-chloroform mixture followed by ethanol precipitation. Silica and anion exchange based techniques utilize DNA binding media that is in the form of membranes or solid phase such as spin columns. Many commercial DNA isolation kits are available in the market. The kits use varying protocols and the time for nucleic acid isolation can range from a few minutes to few hours depending on the protocol that has been used in the kit. The kits typically contain all the required solvents and buffers.26 Numerous studies have been done to compare various kits based on hands-on- time, cost per DNA isolation, ease of use, the yield and quality. However, when setting up a new project, it is always advisable to evaluate different kits for their suitability for the sample of interest from which DNA is to be isolated.16

2.4.1 Solution based extraction techniques

The most common solution based extraction technique is the phenol-chloroform based method which has been extensively used with great success. The phenol-chloroform extraction technique depends on phase separation. The lysed samples are mixed with a phenol-chloroform solution where DNA or RNA partitions in the aqueous phase depending on the pH and salt concentrations of the solutions. If the solution is neutral or basic, RNA partitions in the organic phase or in the interface together with proteins, while DNA partitions in the aqueous phase. Centrifugation is done to separate the two phases and residual phenol can be removed by extracting the purified sample using chloroform. The procedure is completed by precipitating the nucleic acid from the aqueous phase using ethanol. This technique is inexpensive, however, it involves the use of phenol which is toxic. The presence of residual phenol in the extracted DNA can impact negatively on downstream analysis that may involve the use of enzymes. Phenol is neurotoxic and can cause severe burns and therefore care must be taken when using it.[27]

2.4.2 Silica based extraction techniques

The silica based techniques that are used by most current methods offer a fast and robust method for DNA purification. This technique is dependent on the simple fact that DNA adsorbs onto silica surfaces in the presence of high concentrations of chaotropic salts. The silica can be in the form of two different formats: particles that are coated on magnetic beads or silica columns. Many commercial kits using the silica based technique are available, some of which are automated. The buffers used in cell lysis can be chosen in such a manner that during adsorption, only DNA adsorbs onto the silica while all other biomolecules such as RNA and proteins remain in solution. Cellular debris and other biomolecules are washed out using ethanol while the DNA is retained on the silica surface. The DNA is eluted using low salt buffer such as Tris-EDTA (TE) or water. Relatively pure DNA can be obtained using silica based technique; however, treatment of the purified DNA with RNase to remove residual RNA may sometimes be helpful. Care should be taken to wash out all the ethanol to make sure that it does not interfere with downstream applications e.g. presence of ethanol in DNA samples can cause the sample to "float" out of gel electrophoresis wells causing a loss of sample.[28]

2.4.3 Anion exchange chromatography

This purification method relies on the interaction between the negatively charged phosphate backbone of DNA and positively charged functional groups found on an anion exchange resin. The sample is loaded under low salt concentration to allow DNA to bind. A medium strength buffer is used to wash off RNA, proteins and other cellular metabolites. The DNA is then eluted using high strength buffer. Additionally, alcohol precipitation can be used for desalting as well as concentrating the isolated DNA. Since the DNA is eluted with high salt buffer, most downstream applications will require the sample to be desalted. Plasmid DNA is routinely precipitated with ethanol; however, ethanol precipitation of genomic DNA makes it harder to be redissolved. If desalting or concentration of genomic DNA is required, it is best done using isopropanol precipitation or desalting columns.[29]

2.5 Characterization of isolated DNA

Because DNA absorbs at 260nm while protein absorbs at 280 nm, the UV absorbance ratio at A_{260}/A_{280} is generally accepted as a measure of the nucleic acid purity from the contamination of any cellular proteins. A ratio of 1.8 and above is considered as good quality. Organic compounds and chaotropic salts usually absorb at 230nm and therefore the A_{260}/A_{230} ratio can be used to evaluate the presence of residual contaminants from the extraction of DNA. A value of 1.5 and above is considered to be good. A measure of turbidity at 320nm can also be used to evaluate presence of contaminants. The quality of DNA can be assessed by using gel electrophoresis, which provides valuable information on the integrity of isolated DNA. More vigorous isolation techniques can lead to degradation of DNA, which is evident on the gel as a smear of low molecular weight DNA.[30] DNA quality can also be characterized by using the Agilent 2100 analyzer[31] or real time polymerase chain reaction (qPCR).[32] DNA quantitation is commonly done by UV absorbance. Spectrophotometers such as the NanoDrop developed by NanoDrop Technologies are capable of utilizing as little as one microliter of sample for absorbance measurements with a large dynamic range spanning three orders of magnitude. Usually the conversion factors for 1 absorbance unit at 260nm are 50μg/mL for double stranded DNA, 33μg/mL for single stranded DNA, and 20-30μg/mL for oligonucleotides. Although most quantification work on nucleic acids is done using UV absorbance, this method has some sensitivity and accuracy limits. A_{260} measurements can be altered by contaminants such as free nucleotides leading to erroneous quantification. Fluorescent dyes that selectively bind DNA have also been used for the characterization DNA. In spite of the fact that fluorescent dyes are more expensive than using UV absorbance techniques, the benefits of using fluorescent dyes outweighs their cost drawback. The dyes have a high affinity for DNA and exhibit increased fluorescence enhancement after binding. This enables quantification of very small amounts of DNA. The sensitivity can be more than 10,000 times greater than UV absorbance measurements. Furthermore, a great advantage of fluorescent dyes over UV is that measurements are not affected by the presence of free nucleotides or proteins. Commonly used dyes include PicoGreen and OliGreen for DNA.

2.6 Potential pitfalls of DNA isolation

Residual cellular RNA can be found in the samples of isolated DNA. This is more common when samples are from organs that exhibit more transcriptional activities such as the tissue samples of liver or kidney. Since RNA also absorbs UV light at 260 nm, the presence of any RNA in DNA samples adversely affect the quantitative UV measurements. The presence of RNA in isolated DNA samples also interferes with sequencing and reduces the efficiency of amplification. RNA contamination can be eliminated by treating the sample with RNase to degrade the RNA. The presence of proteins in isolated DNA samples can be the result of incomplete digestion by proteases and interfere with the mobility of DNA during gel electrophoresis as well as altering the kinetics of other enzymatic reactions. Residual organic solvents such as ethanol, phenol, chloroform etc. will negatively affect most downstream procedures while salts will slow down or inhibit enzymatic activity such as restriction enzymes. Furthermore, just because a sample contains only DNA is not absolute proof of good quality. This is because during isolation, the sample can be contaminated with DNA from other sources. Such external DNA will give a false impression during DNA quantitation and interfere with amplification procedures.[33]

2.7 RNA isolation techniques

Total RNA can be divided into several groups of RNA which include messenger RNA (mRNA), transfer RNA (tRNA), ribosomal RNA (rRNA), mitochondrial RNA (mtRNA) and many groups of small RNA such as microRNA (miRNA), and piwi-interacting RNA (piRNA). On average, about 80% of total RNA is made up of rRNA while 1-5% is mRNA. Expression of mRNA can vary greatly from cell to cell and can range from a few copies per cell to several thousand.[34] If poly-adenylated mRNA is required, it is preferably isolated from total RNA by capturing the poly(A) tail onto oligo(dT) primers. The same approach can also be used to isolate mRNA directly from the lysate without necessarily isolating the total RNA. Similar to the isolation of DNA, the requirements for both quality and quantity of isolated RNA would determine the choice of isolation method. For example, RNA isolated for use in microarrays and RT-PCR needs to be of high purity and free from contaminants such as salts, phenol, ethanol etc. whereas methods such as Northern blotting may be more forgiving for contaminants. When purifying RNA, it is very important that it is prevented from degradation by both endogenous and exogenous RNases. Many commercial kits for RNA isolation have been developed, some of them are designed to isolate specific group of RNA, e.g. mRNA.

The most common solution based technique for RNA isolation is the guanidinium, phenol-chloroform ethanol precipitation. This technique was first reported by Chomczynski and Sacchi in 1987 and later revisited in 2006 by the same authors.[35] Over time, the method has been widely used and modified. Basically, it operates on the principle that RNA can be separated from DNA if an acidic solution containing sodium acetate, phenol, chloroform and guanidinium isothiocyanate is used. Guanidinium isothiocyanate is a very effective protein denaturant and when used in buffers, it provides an RNase-free environment. Phenol dissociates nucleic acids from proteins while chloroform denatures both proteins and lipids. Chloroform also makes nucleic acids less soluble in phenol and maintains the separation of the aqueous and the organic layer. Mixing the lysate with the acidic solution results in phase separation with the RNA partitioning in the upper aqueous layer while the DNA, lipids and protein remain either in the interphase or in the lower organic phenol layer. The upper aqueous layer is retrieved and the total RNA recovered through precipitation with isopropanol.

2.7.1 Sequence specific RNA isolation

To capture RNA whose sequence is known, biotinylated DNA probes consisting of a sequence complimentary to the known portion of the RNA to be isolated can be used. The probe-RNA complex is then isolated using streptavidin coated magnetic beads through the interaction of biotin and streptavidin. The beads are pulled out of solution using a magnet, and the supernatant containing cellular debris and contaminants is removed. The captured RNA is then eluted from the beads for downstream applications.[36]

2.7.2 Isolation of mRNA

To isolate mRNA, a sample containing total RNA is loaded in an oligo(dT) spin column. In high salt conditions, the 3′ poly(dA) tail of mRNA hybridize to oligo(dT) that have been immobilized on the column. The contaminants are washed off with a high salt buffer and a low salt buffer. The mRNA is then eluted using a low ionic strength buffer. Alternatively, magnetic beads coated with poly(dT) beads can be added to total RNA sample. The beads are captured with a magnet and the contaminants are removed. The bead complex is then washed and mRNA are eluted. This technique is also useful for concentrating mRNA samples.[37]

2.7.3 Isolation of Small RNA with <200 nucleotides (nt)

The most widely used techniques for total RNA isolation are phenol or silica based. These methods were designed and optimized for isolation of high molecular weight RNA because small RNA molecules were thought to be unimportant. As such, these traditional methods do not retain most of the small RNA fraction and are therefore not suitable for the isolation of small RNA (<200nt). Since small RNA only makes up a small fraction of total RNA, the use of total RNA as starting material for any detection method can potentially lower its sensitivity and/or specificity. Small RNA such as microRNA, siRNA, piwiRNA, rasiRNA and others have been shown to perform important biological functions. In order to isolate these RNA, the traditional methods have been redesigned or completely new methods have been developed. Initially, separation and enrichment of small RNA from total RNA was done by size fractionation using size exclusion columns or by using 12-15% denaturing polyacrylamide gel electrophoresis. These techniques however only yield minute amounts of small RNA. The need to isolate larger amounts of small RNA has led to development of the new methods. Commercially available kits for small RNA isolation include PureLink from Invitrogen (Carlsbad, CA, USA)38, miRNeasy Mini Kit from Qiagen (Valencia, CA, USA)39 and mirVana that is produced and sold by Ambion (Austin, Texas, USA)40 among others. The mirVana kit makes use of organic as well as solid phase isolation. RNA is first isolated from the lysed sample using acidic phenol-chloroform solution that separates RNA from proteins, DNA and other cellular debris. The isolated RNA can be further purified for small RNA by immobilizing them onto a glass-fiber filter. A low ionic strength buffer is used to wash the filter before small RNA is eluted with a relatively low ethanol concentration (25%).[41]

2.8 Characterization of isolated RNA

Similar to the characterization of isolated DNA, the traditional method for the quantification of RNA is by using UV absorbance measurements. A diluted sample of RNA is measured at 260 and 280nm. Using the Beer-Lambert law which assumes that the relationship between absorbance and concentration is linear, the concentration of RNA can be calculated. An absorbance of 1.0 using A_{260} measurement translates to an RNA concentration of ~40μg/mL. The A_{260}/A_{280} ratio is used as a measure of RNA purity since proteins absorb at A_{280}. A ratio of 1.82:1 is accepted as a measure of highly purified RNA. In the presence of DNA contamination, UV measurements can overestimate the RNA concentration because DNA also absorbs at 260nm, however, if DNA contamination is suspected, the sample should be treated with RNase-free DNase to eliminate the DNA. The quantity of RNA can be determined by using fluorescent dyes such as RiboGreen and fluorometric measurements. This method is less sensitive to free nucleotides and proteins but can be inaccurate in the presence of DNA contamination. The integrity of isolated RNA is often measured by using denaturing gel electrophoresis. When total RNA sample is run on a denaturing gel stained with ethidium bromide, the 28S and 18S rRNA show up as intense bands. The 28S and 18S rRNA band intensity ratio can be used as a measure of the integrity of RNA. A ratio of 2:1 (28S:18S) is usually accepted as a measure of intact RNA. Smeared 28S and 18S coupled with a ratio below 2:1 is an indication of RNA degradation. Highly degraded RNA samples appear as a smear in the region of low molecular weight. For limited amounts of RNA samples, other RNA staining dyes that are more sensitive such as SYBR Gold and SYBR Green can be used.[42] A more recent method is the Agilent 2100 Bioanalyzer that uses a microfluidics-based platform in conjunction with capillary electrophoresis and fluorescent dyes to perform both qualitative and quantitative measurements. The sample size for the 2100 Bioanalyzer can be as low as 1μL of 10ng/μL RNA.[43]

2.9 Potential pitfalls of RNA isolation

The presence of RNase causes degradation of RNA and will affect all downstream applications that require intact RNA. The presence of polysaccharides especially in liver and muscle tissues can affect RNA isolation and lead to low yields. Polysaccharides also inhibit RT-PCR, though, the mechanism of interference is not known. Residual genomic DNA in isolated RNA interferes with RT-PCR, microarrays and even nuclease protection experiments. The DNA contaminants can compete for PCR primers or other probes for the detection of RNA and lead to false positive signals. DNA is easily removed from the isolated RNA by digesting it with DNase. The DNase can be easily removed before downstream experiments are performed. Residual EDTA and solvents used to isolate RNA can chelate Mg2+ ions that are needed by polymerases in PCR and prevent cDNA synthesis. They can also interfere with microarray experiments. Carryover salts from buffers and other solutions slow down reverse transcriptase and cDNA synthesis. Alcohol, chloroform and phenol that may be carried over during isolation affect most biological experiments by inhibiting enzymatic activity.

3. Detection and quantificaton of DNA adducts

Referring to Figure 3, depending upon the type of biological samples, nucleic acid adducts can exist at the genomic level (i.e. intact DNA) or individual nucleotide adducts, which result from biodegradation and have been excreted into biofluids (e.g. urine).

For the analysis of genomic DNA, the majority of developed methods require breaking down the genomic DNA into monomeric nucleotides or dinucleotides. This can be accomplished by either chemical hydrolysis or enzymatic digestion as shown in the schematic diagram in Figure 3. With the chemical hydrolysis of genomic DNA, if an acidic compound is used, it may induce the depurination of DNA and/or the hydrolysis of DNA adducts. Thus, the alternative enzymatic approach is more widely used to digest genomic DNA. To ensure a complete digestion of genomic DNA, a combination of different nucleases, for instance exonuclease and endonuclease, is often used. Following the digestion of genomic DNA, the approach for analyzing DNA adducts is the same for all types of biological samples, i.e. DNA adducts are separated from a mixture of nucleotides prior to their specific detection.

The removal of unmodified nucleotides can greatly enhance the specificity of the subsequent detection of DNA adducts. This is because, in many studies, the ratio of unmodified nucleotides to nucleotide adducts can be as high as 10^{12} : 1. As indicated in Figure 3, the separation of DNA adducts is usually achieved by using one or a combination of chromatographic techniques. Often times, this part of an experimental procedure for analyzing specific DNA adducts is referred as enrichment of DNA adducts or a solid-phase extraction of DNA adducts. After the separation of DNA adducts, there are a number of different analytical techniques that have been chosen for carrying out the end point measurements of specific DNA adducts as shown in Figure 3. In general, the end point measurements can be divided into two groups, namely with or without the use of reporting labels. The use of reporting labels, for instance ^{32}P radioactive isotope, can achieve lower limit of detection (LOD). On the other hand, the direct adduct measurements, i.e. without the use of any reporting labels, can achieve higher specificity and also allow the molecular structure of adducts to be determined. The selection of a specific analytical technique is ultimately determined by the physiochemical properties of DNA adduct and its abundance in the biological samples. More details on each analytical technique that have been used to detect DNA adducts are covered in subsections 3.1.1 to 3.1.5. Readers are advised that the aim of this section is to provide an overview of the current methodologies for DNA adduct analysis that have been used in the last five years and is not intended to cover all the reports in the literature. Several excellent reviews on the detection of specific DNA adducts are available in the literature.[44,45]

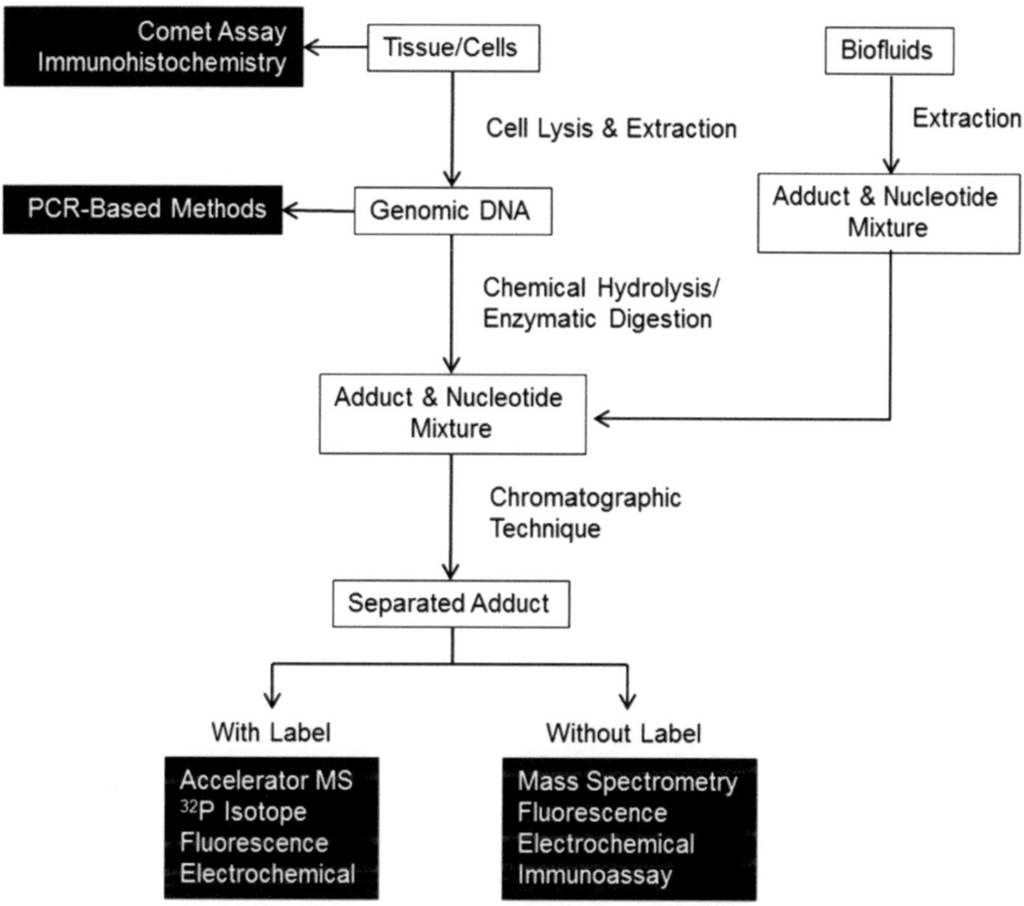

Fig. 3. Schematic diagram of different approaches for analyzing DNA adduction.

It is important to realize that the digestion of genomic DNA into its monomeric nucleotides is equivalent to erasing all the DNA sequence information, thus the locations of adduction within the genome can no longer be determined. In order to determine the locations of DNA adduction, genomic DNA has to be analyzed. There are a number of polymerase chain reaction (PCR) based methods that have been developed which allow us to determine the locations of adduction. In general, these methodologies rely on using specific enzymatic activities or chemical hydrolysis methods to create unique reaction products that correspond to each location of DNA adduct. For instance, an adduct-containing DNA fragment can be cleaved at or near the adduct by a DNA repair enzyme. The resulting fragments are amplified by using PCR. By sequencing the PCR amplicons, the locations of adduct can then be determined. With the use of PCR, very small amounts of starting material are required. However, the drawbacks of this approach include the specificity of the methods for breaking down the genomic DNA at or near the location of an adduct, the lack of information on the adduct identity, and the inability to determine the location of adducts that are close or next to each other. Overall, the PCR-based methods are the only approach that can be used to determine the location of adducts but may not be universally applicable.

With a wide variety of DNA adductions, there is no single method that can be used to analyze every possible DNA adduct. Before spending time and efforts to develop and/or validate a method, the extent of DNA damage can be evaluated by a non-specific method called comet assay. As indicated in Figure 3, the starting materials for comet assay are tissue or cellular samples. In the comet assay, cells are first embedded in an agarose gel. The cells are then lysed under a condition that induces DNA to supercoil and link to the nucleus matrix. With the presence of DNA damage, it is easier to electrophoretically pull the DNA out from the cell nucleus. By using microscopic fluorometry to monitor the migration of DNA, which forms a tail resembling a comet, the extent of cellular DNA damage can be evaluated. The higher the fluorescence intensity in the tail, the higher the extent of DNA damage. Alternatively, for determining the presence of DNA adducts on a tissue section, the approach of immunohistochemistry can be used, providing a specific detection antibody against the adduct of interest is available.

3.1 Accelerated Mass Spectrometry (AMS)

AMS has generally been regarded as the most sensitive method available in the detection of DNA adducts with a limit of detection (LOD) ranging from ~1-10 adducts per 10^{12} nucleotides.[46] In AMS, the abundance of specific radioisotopes is measured. For measuring biological samples, the most relevant isotopes are ^{14}C and ^{3}H. The sensitivity of AMS is high enough that even very small amounts of exogenously applied radioisotopes can be detected, thereby allowing AMS to be used in human studies.[47] The sample preparation protocol involves the extraction of cellular DNA which can be either analyzed as intact DNA or subjected to enzymatic digestion into nucleotides. This is followed by the separation with HPLC to isolate the adduct of interest. Sample analysis usually involves combustion into elemental carbon or CO_2 for ^{14}C or titanium hydride for ^{3}H. However despite the aforementioned advantages, AMS has several disadvantages as well. Before the adduct measurements, the subject or host has to be exposed to radioactive isotopic-labeled precursors. As such, biomonitoring studies are often prohibited. Since the chemical structure of the adduct is lost due to its decomposition into the elemental components, there is a requirement to compare the chromatograms of synthetic adducts (if available) with that of the sample, to accurately identify the adduct. Significant emphasis must be placed on sample purity to prevent the false positive signals from any radioactive background noise. Currently, there are a limited number (5-10) of AMS spectrometers worldwide that are specifically setup for biological sample analysis.[48] To increase the viability to analyze samples from humans in terms of possible exposure to unlabeled carcinogenic/genotoxic compounds, postlabeling methods have been developed to derivatize DNA adducts of interest with ^{14}C or ^{3}H isotopes.[46]

3.2 ^{32}P radioisotope labeling

The ^{32}P-postlabeling method is useful in analyzing a vast array of DNA adducts (e.g. polycyclic aromatic hydrocarbons, aromatic amines, etc.) and is also highly regarded with respect to sensitivity (LOD of 1 adduct/10^{10} nucleotides). Following the isolation of genomic DNA, the sample is enzymatically digested into 3′-mononucleotides or less commonly dinucleotides. Enrichment procedures call for the use of either immunoaffinity chromatography or *n*-butanol as a means to extract adduct from unmodified nucleotides. The extracted nucleotide adduct is then dephosphorylated using nuclease P1 treatment. Phosphorylation (or ^{32}P-postlabeling) is then performed by the specific activity of T-4 polynucleotide kinases. This produces 3′,5′-bisphosphates which are subsequently separated by using a chromatographic technique such as high performance liquid chromatography (HPLC), two-dimensional thin layer chromatography (2D-TLC), or gel separation. Resolution is greater for HPLC but sensitivity is lower than

TLC. Thus, for quantitative analysis, TLC is more common. The initial standardization protocols for quantitation purposes in the 1990s were found to be only qualitative. More recently, a method that overcame some of the shortcomings of earlier trials was reported.[49] With efficient isolation of DNA adduct and labeling, quantitation of specific adducts is possible. A set of standardized protocols are now instituted and allow quantitation of several types of DNA adducts (aromatic amines, PAHs, methylating agents).[50] Nevertheless, the required large quantities of radioactive isotopes and the lengthy time necessary for completing the labeling procedure are problematic. Also, structural characterization of DNA adduct is not possible, thus rigorous co-chromatography against synthetic or previously identified adducts is required to identify DNA adducts.

3.3 Mass spectrometry

With the advances in mass spectrometry, the applications of mass spectrometry to analyze DNA adducts have continued to grow in the recent years. A number of excellent reviews have been published.[51] Following the isolation and digestion of genomic DNA, the analysis of DNA adducts can be carried out by using either gas chromatography-mass spectrometry (GC-MS) or liquid chromatography-mass spectrometry (LC-MS). In the case of GC-MS, the less volatile adducts have to be derivatized prior to the GC-MS measurements. Also, owing to the thermal decomposition, the analysis of adducts are often limited to nucleobases. With the development of soft ionization techniques like electrospray ionization (ESI) and matrix-assisted laser desorption/ionization (MALDI), liquid chromatography has been successfully coupled to mass spectrometry. This allows the accurate mass of specific adducts to be measured as well as their molecular structure can be determined by using tandem mass spectrometry (MS/MS). Specifically, following the elution of an adduct from a LC column and the ionization of adduct, the precursor (or parent) ion of the adduct is selected by the first mass analyzer. The precursor ion is then fragmented by a process called collision-induced dissociation (CID). After that, all the fragment ions which originated from the selected adduct are separated and detected in the second mass analyzer. The molecular structure of selected adduct including the type and position of adduction can be determined with high accuracy by analyzing the MS/MS data. The structural information is very desirable as it may provide insight into the metabolism of a genotoxic agent before adduction. Additionally, small sample sizes are possible with the LC-MS method. This is in contrast to other methodologies for determining molecular structures, such as nuclear magnetic resonance (NMR) spectroscopy which requires larger sample sizes and higher concentration of adduct. For the quantitation of adducts, the choice of instrumentation is a mass spectrometer that is equipped with a triple quadrupole mass analyzer. To ensure sufficient high sensitivity is achieved, nano-electrospray ionization and/or the selected reaction monitoring (SRM) mode in a triple quadrupole mass spectrometer are recommended. Recently, a two-dimensional linear quadrupole ion trap mass spectrometer operating in a constant neutral loss scanning mode with subsequent triple stage MS was utilized in the detection and quantitation of five different DNA adducts.[52] This technique was demonstrated to be capable of screening various carcinogenic adducts at low LOD (~1 adduct per 10^8 nucleotides) with small quantities of DNA (~10 μg). This is an order of magnitude more sensitive than the best available immunoassays and close to that of ^{32}P-postlabeling method. Several reports have been published in which ESI MS has been coupled to capillary electrophoresis (CE) or nanoLC, thereby providing the capability to examine adducts at low levels. For example, an LOD of ~5 adducts per 10^9nucleosides with a linear dynamic range between 70 amol and 70 fmol has recently been reported.[53]

3.4 Fluorometric and electrochemical detection

Following the chromatographic separation of adducts, their detection can be achieved by fluorescence, electrochemical (EC), or electron capture detection (ECD) providing the adducts have either intrinsic or chemically induced properties to generate the corresponding signals. In general, the sensitivity of these techniques are often in the range of 1-10 adducts per 10^8 nucleotides and require ~20-100 μg of genomic sample. If pure standards are available, structural characterization as well as the quantitation of adducts are possible. However, the number of adducts which have the required intrinsic physiochemical properties are limited. Also, the derivatization (or labeling) of adducts which lack the intrinsic properties to generate the corresponding signals is labor intensive and the yield is usually low. These techniques have been used to detect adducts with inherent fluorescence property (e.g. PAH and aflatoxin B_1) or electrochemical characteristics (e.g. 8-oxo-7,8-dihydroguanine). Providing the adduct has a derivatizable group in comparison to unmodified DNA, the derivatization of adduct with a volatile ligand, such as pentafluorophenyl, would allow the use of GC which is coupled to an electron capture detector, whose sensitivity can be as low as zeptomole.[54] Similar sensitivity can also be achieved by using laser induced fluorescence (LIF) providing the phosphate group of a nucleotide containing the adduct has been derivatized with an appropriate fluorophore.

3.5 Immunoassay

As mentioned earlier, antibodies can be used to detect DNA adducts in a wide variety of tissue samples (immunohistochemistry). The same antibody can be applied to the detection of digested or excreted DNA adducts in various biofluids by using an enzyme linked immunosorbent assay (ELISA) assay or an equivalent immunoassay. Various antibodies against adducts with either high or low molecular weight are available. However, in clinical studies, the specificity of antibodies to recognize adducts is relatively poor. This is partly due to the fact that DNA adducts are not separated from the other unmodified nucleotides or cellular components before being measured by immunoassay. To address this technical issue, trapped in agarose DNA immunostaining (TARDIS) assay has been developed. An extensive review of this topic has been discussed.[55] In general, monoclonal antibodies are preferred over polyclonal antibodies with regards to specificity but polyclonal antibodies can provide higher sensitivity (1 adduct per 10^8 nucleotides). The overall assay sensitivity is dependent on the affinity of antibody for the adduct of interest and the detectability of reporting label being used.

4. Detection and quantificaton RNA adducts

In comparison to the DNA adduct analysis, the number of reports on RNA adduct analysis are significantly less. This could be partly due to the fact that, unlike the genomic DNA, cellular RNAs are not used as templates to generate any biological molecules. Furthermore, there is a natural turnover of cellular RNA, i.e. the gene expression and degradation of RNA are continuous processes within the cells. Owing to these reasons, the effects of RNA adduction have often been considered to be less important than DNA adduction. Nevertheless, RNA adduction has been associated with different diseases which include cancer. The same methods that have been used to detect DNA adducts can also be applied to the detection and quantification of RNA adducts. To ensure higher specificity is achieved, it is important to remove any genomic DNA from cellular RNA samples prior to the RNA adduct analysis. As mentioned earlier in this chapter, the most effective approach to remove genomic DNA is by carrying out the DNase digestion, and the intact cellular RNA that remains in the sample can be easily purified by using one of the standard RNA purification methods. After that, cellular RNA is ready to be digested into nucleotides, unless the information on the location of RNA adducts is desired. To determine the location of adducts within an RNA fragment, the PCR-based methods can be used. For instance, reverse transcriptase would prematurely stop the cDNA synthesis at the adduct location and produce a template which is unique to the adduct location for the subsequent PCR reaction. In general, the PCR-based methods have lower specificity than those methods that have been developed to analyze a mixture of nucleotides including RNA adducts.

5. References

[1] Preston, R. J.; Ross, J. A., DNA-Reactive Agents. In *Comprehensive Toxicology*, Charlene, A. M., Ed. Elsevier: Oxford, 2010; pp 349-360.

[2] Cohen, S. M.; Arnold, L. L., Chemical carcinogenesis. *Toxicol. Sci.* 2011, *120*, S76-S92.

[3] Alekseyev, Y. O.; Romano, L. J., Effects of benzo[a]pyrene adduct stereochemistry on downstream DNA replication in vitro: evidence for different adduct conformations within the active site of DNA polymerase I (Klenow fragment). *Biochemistry* 2002, *41*, 4467-4479.

[4] Schmitz, O. J., Analysis of DNA modifications. *Anal Bioanal Chem* 2006, *384* (1), 34-6.

[5] Turesky, R. J.; Vouros, P., Formation and analysis of heterocyclic aromatic amine-DNA adducts in vitro and in vivo. *J Chromatogr B Analyt Technol Biomed Life Sci* 2004, *802* (1), 155-66.

[6] Farmer, P. B.; Brown, K.; Tompkins, E.; Emms, V. L.; Jones, D. J.; Singh, R.; Phillips, D. H., DNA adducts: mass spectrometry methods and future prospects. *Toxicol Appl Pharmacol* 2005, *207* (2 Suppl), 293-301.

[7] Banoub, J. H.; Limbach, P. A.; Editors, *Mass Spectrometry Of Nucleosides And Nucleic Acids*. CRC Press: 2010; p 492 pp.

[8] Sar, D. G.; Montes-Bayon, M.; Blanco-Gonzalez, E.; Sanz-Medel, A., Quantitative methods for studying DNA interactions with chemotherapeutic cisplatin. *TrAC, Trends Anal. Chem.* 2010, *29*, 1390-1398.

[9] Koivisto, P.; Peltonen, K., Analytical methods in DNA and protein adduct analysis. *Anal. Bioanal. Chem.* 2010, *398*, 2563-2572.

[10] Tan, S. C.; Yiap, B. C., DNA, RNA, and protein extraction: the past and the present. *J Biomed Biotechnol* 2009, *2009*, 574398; Tan, S. C.; Yiap, B. C., DNA, RNA, and protein extraction: the past and the present. *J. Biomed. Biotechnol.* 2009 , No pp. given.

[11] GEHealthcare, Nucleic Acid Sample Preparation for Downstream Analyses. GE Healthcare Bio-Sciences Corp: www.gelifesciences.com, 2009; Vol. 28-9624-00.

[12] Psifidi, A.; Dovas, C. I.; Banos, G., A comparison of six methods for genomic DNA extraction suitable for PCR-based genotyping applications using ovine milk samples. *Molecular and Cellular Probes* 2010, *24* (2), 93-98.

[13] Nocker, A.; Camper, A. K., Novel approaches toward preferential detection of viable cells using nucleic acid amplification techniques. *FEMS Microbiol Lett* 2009, *291* (2), 137-42.

[14] Hansen, W. L.; Bruggeman, C. A.; Wolffs, P. F., Evaluation of new preanalysis sample treatment tools and DNA isolation protocols to improve bacterial pathogen detection in whole blood. *J Clin Microbiol* 2009, *47* (8), 2629-31.

[15] Wong, H. Y.; Lim, E. S.; Tan-Siew, W. F., Amplification volume reduction on DNA database samples using FTA™ Classic Cards. *Forensic Sci Int Genet* 2011.

[16] Mackay, I. M.; Editor, *Real-Time PCR in Microbiology: From Diagnosis to Characterization.* Caister Academic Press: 2007; p 454 pp.

[17] Miller, D. N.; Bryant, J. E.; Madsen, E. L.; Ghiorse, W. C., Evaluation and optimization of DNA extraction and purification procedures for soil and sediment samples. *Appl Environ Microbiol* 1999, *65* (11), 4715-24.

[18] Tran, M. Q. T.; Nygren, Y.; Lundin, C.; Naredi, P.; Bjoern, E., Evaluation of cell lysis methods for platinum metallomic studies of human malignant cells. *Anal. Biochem.* 2010, *396*, 76-82.

[19] Vandeventer, P. E.; Weigel, K. M.; Salazar, J.; Erwin, B.; Irvine, B.; Doebler, R.; Nadim, A.; Cangelosi, G. A.; Niemz, A., Mechanical disruption of lysis-resistant bacterial cells by use of a miniature, low-power, disposable device. *J Clin Microbiol* 2011, *49* (7), 2533-9.

[20] Lin, Z.; Cai, Z., Cell lysis methods for high-throughput screening or miniaturized assays. *Biotechnol J* 2009, *4* (2), 210-5.

[21] Klimek-Ochab, M.; Brzezińska-Rodak, M.; Zymańczyk-Duda, E.; Lejczak, B.; Kafarski, P., Comparative study of fungal cell disruption--scope and limitations of the methods. *Folia Microbiol (Praha)* 2011, *56* (5), 469-75.

[22] Coombs, N. J.; Gough, A. C.; Primrose, J. N., Optimisation of DNA and RNA extraction from archival formalin-fixed tissue. *Nucleic Acids Res* 1999, *27* (16), e12.

[23] Leuko, S.; Goh, F.; Ibanez-Peral, R.; Burns, B. P.; Walter, M. R.; Neilan, B. A., Lysis efficiency of standard DNA extraction methods for Halococcus spp. in an organic rich environment. *Extremophiles* 2008, *12* (Copyright (C) 2011 U.S. National Library of Medicine.), 301-8.

[24] Queipo-Ortuño, M. I.; Tena, F.; Colmenero, J. D.; Morata, P., Comparison of seven commercial DNA extraction kits for the recovery of Brucella DNA from spiked human serum samples using real-time PCR. *Eur J Clin Microbiol Infect Dis* 2008, *27* (2), 109-14.

[25] McGinley, J. N.; Zhu, Z.; Jiang, W.; Thompson, H. J., Collection of epithelial cells from rodent mammary gland via laser capture microdissection yielding high-quality RNA suitable for microarray analysis. *Biol Proced Online* 2010, *12* (1), 9026.

[26] Muñoz-Cadavid, C.; Rudd, S.; Zaki, S. R.; Patel, M.; Moser, S. A.; Brandt, M. E.; Gómez, B. L., Improving molecular detection of fungal DNA in formalin-fixed paraffin-embedded tissues: comparison of five tissue DNA extraction methods using panfungal PCR. *J Clin Microbiol* 2010, *48* (6), 2147-53.

[27] Farrugia, A.; Keyser, C.; Ludes, B., Efficiency evaluation of a DNA extraction and purification protocol on archival formalin-fixed and paraffin-embedded tissue. *Forensic Sci. Int.* 2010, *194*, e25-e28.

[28] Lee, H. Y.; Park, M. J.; Kim, N. Y.; Sim, J. E.; Yang, W. I.; Shin, K. J., Simple and highly effective DNA extraction methods from old skeletal remains using silica columns. *Forensic Sci Int Genet* 2010, *4* (5), 275-80.

[29] Sandhu, J.; Kaur, B.; Armstrong, C.; Talbot, C. J.; Steward, W. P.; Farmer, P. B.; Singh, R., Determination of 5-methyl-2'-deoxycytidine in genomic DNA using high performance liquid chromatography-ultraviolet detection. *J. Chromatogr., B: Anal. Technol. Biomed. Life Sci.* 2009, *877*, 1957-1961.

[30] Clements, D. N.; Wood, S.; Carter, S. D.; Ollier, W. E., Assessment of the quality and quantity of genomic DNA recovered from canine blood samples by three different extraction methods. *Res Vet Sci* 2008, *85* (1), 74-9.

[31] Gorzkiewicz, M.; Duleba, A.; Rychlicka, E.; Wozniak, M.; Grzybowski, T.; Sliwka, K., Evaluation of the Agilent 2100 Bioanalyzer as a tool for DNA analysis in forensic genetics. *Z Zagadnien Nauk Sadowych* 2010, *81*, 91-100.

[32] Bhat, S.; Curach, N.; Mostyn, T.; Bains, G. S.; Griffiths, K. R.; Emslie, K. R., Comparison of methods for accurate quantification of DNA mass concentration with traceability to the international system of units. *Anal Chem* 2010, *82* (17), 7185-92.

[33] Singh, R.; Teichert, F.; Verschoyle, R. D.; Kaur, B.; Vives, M.; Sharma, R. A.; Steward, W. P.; Gescher, A. J.; Farmer, P. B., Simultaneous determination of 8-oxo-2'-deoxyguanosine and 8-oxo-2'-deoxyadenosine in DNA using online column-switching liquid chromatography/tandem mass spectrometry. *Rapid Commun Mass Spectrom* 2009, *23* (1), 151-60.

[34] Zhdanov, V. P., Conditions of appreciable influence of microRNA on a large number of target mRNAs. *Mol Biosyst* 2009, *5* (6), 638-43.

[35] Chomczynski, P.; Sacchi, N., Single-step method of RNA isolation by acid guanidinium thiocyanate-phenol-chloroform extraction. *Anal. Biochem.* 1987, *162*, 156-9.

[36] Suzuki, T., Chaplet column chromatography: isolation of a large set of individual RNAs in a single step. *Methods Enzymol* 2007, *425*, 231-9.

[37] Saiyed, Z.; Telang, S.; Ramchand, C., Application of magnetic techniques in the field of drug discovery and biomedicine. *Biomagn Res Technol* 2003, *1* (1), 2.

[38] Zhou, Q. J.; Xiang, L. X.; Shao, J. Z.; Hu, R. Z.; Lu, Y. L.; Yao, H.; Dai, L. C., In vitro differentiation of hepatic progenitor cells from mouse embryonic stem cells induced by sodium butyrate. *J Cell Biochem* 2007, *100* (1), 29-42.

[39] Nam, D.; Ni, C. W.; Rezvan, A.; Suo, J.; Budzyn, K.; Llanos, A.; Harrison, D. G.; Giddens, D. P.; Jo, H., A model of disturbed flow-induced atherosclerosis in mouse carotid artery by partial ligation and a simple method of RNA isolation from carotid endothelium. *J Vis Exp* 2010, (40).

[40] Sarver, A. L.; Li, L.; Subramanian, S., MicroRNA miR-183 functions as an oncogene by targeting the transcription factor EGR1 and promoting tumor cell migration. *Cancer Res* 2010, *70* (23), 9570-80.

[41] Ramdas, L.; Giri, U.; Ashorn, C. L.; Coombes, K. R.; El-Naggar, A.; Ang, K. K.; Story, M. D., miRNA expression profiles in head and neck squamous cell carcinoma and adjacent normal tissue. *Head Neck* 2009, *31* (5), 642-54.

[42] Aranda, R.; Dineen, S. M.; Craig, R. L.; Guerrieri, R. A.; Robertson, J. M., Comparison and evaluation of RNA quantification methods using viral, prokaryotic, and eukaryotic RNA over a 10(4) concentration range. *Anal Biochem* 2009, *387* (1), 122-7.

[43] Pfaffl, M. W.; Fleige, S.; Riedmaier, I., Validation of lab-on-chip capillary electrophoresis systems for total RNA quality and quantity control. *Biotechnol. Biotechnol. Equip.* 2008, *22*, 829-834.

[44] Himmelstein, M. W.; Boogaard, P. J.; Cadet, J.; Farmer, P. B.; Kim, J. H.; Martin, E. A.; Persaud, R.; Shuker, D. E., Creating context for the use of DNA adduct data in cancer risk assessment: II. Overview of methods of identification and quantitation of DNA damage. *Crit Rev Toxicol* 2009, *39* (8), 679-94.

[45] Kellner, S.; Burhenne, J.; Helm, M., Detection of RNA modifications. *RNA Biol* 2010, *7* (2), 237-47.

[46] Tompkins, E. M.; Farmer, P. B.; Lamb, J. H.; Jukes, R.; Dingley, K.; Ubick, E.; Turteltaub, K. W.; Martin, E. A.; Brown, K., A novel 14C-postlabeling assay using accelerator mass spectrometry for the detection of O6-methyldeoxy-guanosine adducts. *Rapid Communications in Mass Spectrometry* 2006, *20* (5), 883-891.

[47] Coldwell, K. E.; Cutts, S. M.; Ognibene, T. J.; Henderson, P. T.; Phillips, D. R., Detection of Adriamycin–DNA adducts by accelerator mass spectrometry at clinically relevant Adriamycin concentrations. *Nucleic Acids Research* 2008, *36* (16), e100-e100.

[48] Emami, A.; Dyba, M.; Cheema, A. K.; Pan, J.; Nath, R. G.; Chung, F.-L., Detection of the acrolein-derived cyclic DNA adduct by a quantitative 32P-postlabeling/solid-phase extraction/HPLC method: Blocking its artifact formation with glutathione. *Analytical Biochemistry* 2008, *374* (1), 163-172.

[49] Phillips, D. H.; Arlt, V. M., The 32P-postlabeling assay for DNA adducts. *Nat. Protocols* 2007, *2* (11), 2772-2781.

[50] Phillips, D. H.; Castegnaro, M.; on behalf of the trial, p., Standardization and validation of DNA adduct postlabelling methods: report of interlaboratory trials and production of recommended protocols. *Mutagenesis* 1999, *14* (3), 301-315.

[51] Filip, L. r., Mass Spectrometric Determination of DNA Adducts in Human Carcinogenesis. In *Mass Spectrometry of Nucleosides and Nucleic Acids*, CRC Press: 2009; pp 195-255.

[52] Bessette, E. E.; Goodenough, A. K.; Langouët, S.; Yasa, I.; Kozekov, I. D.; Spivack, S. D.; Turesky, R. J., Screening for DNA Adducts by Data-Dependent Constant Neutral Loss-Triple Stage Mass Spectrometry with a Linear Quadrupole Ion Trap Mass Spectrometer. *Analytical Chemistry* 2008, *81* (2), 809-819.

[53] Randall, K. L.; Argoti, D.; Paonessa, J. D.; Ding, Y.; Oaks, Z.; Zhang, Y.; Vouros, P., An improved liquid chromatography–tandem mass spectrometry method for the quantification of 4-aminobiphenyl DNA adducts in urinary bladder cells and tissues. *Journal of Chromatography A* 2010, *1217* (25), 4135-4143.

[54] van Sittert, N. J.; Boogaard, P. J.; Natarajan, A. T.; Tates, A. D.; Ehrenberg, L. G.; Törnqvist, M. A., Formation of DNA adducts and induction of mutagenic effects in rats following 4 weeks inhalation exposure to ethylene oxide as a basis for cancer risk assessment. *Mutation Research/Fundamental and Molecular Mechanisms of Mutagenesis* 2000, *447* (1), 27-48.

[55] Cowell, I. G.; Tilby, M. J.; Austin, C. A., An overview of the visualisation and quantitation of low and high MW DNA adducts using the trapped in agarose DNA immunostaining (TARDIS) assay. *Mutagenesis* 2011 *26* (2), 253-260.

Section 4

Food and Carcinogens

7

Carcinogen Role of Food by Mycotoxins and Knowledge Gap

Margherita Ferrante, Salvatore Sciacca and Gea Oliveri Conti
University of Catania, Department "G.F. Ingrassia" Hygiene and Public Health, Italy

1. Introduction

In today's world health and safety are among the basic human needs. Ensuring food safety has been a major focus of international and national action over the last decades.

Both, microbiological and chemical risks are of concern. The "World Health Organization" (WHO) has identified as significant sources of food-borne diseases contamination of food and feed by mycotoxins (toxic metabolites of molds) and the contamination of fishery products by phycotoxins (toxins produced by algae).

Despite public health and prevention managers have paid particular attention to mycotoxins, in several areas of the world they are still an important food safety issue (Fig 1).

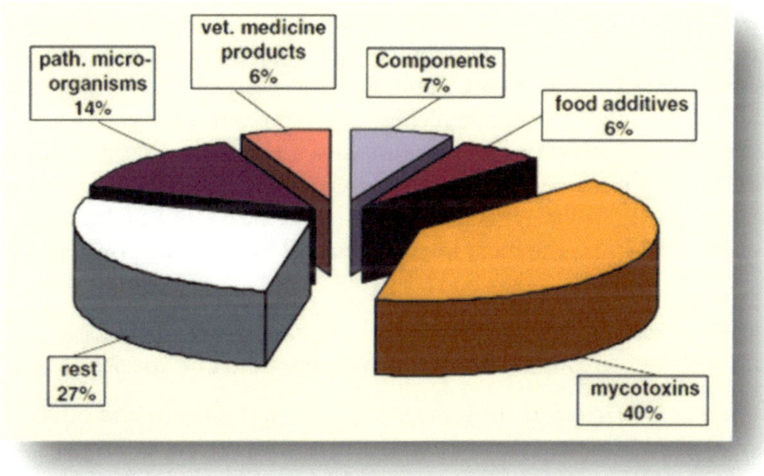

Fig. 1. Notifications for food and feed in 2005 (from EU rapid alert system, by European Commission 2006).

Mycotoxins can cause diseases in humans, crops and animals that have led many Countries to establish limits on mycotoxins in food and feed to safeguard people's health, as well as the economical interests of producers and traders.

The first limits for mycotoxins were set in the late 1960s for the aflatoxins. Already approximately 100 Countries in the world have developed specific limits for mycotoxins in foodstuffs and feedstuffs and their number continues to grow (Van Egmond & Jonker, 2004; WHO, 2002a).

1.1 General information on mycotoxins

The natural fungal flora associated with foods is dominated by four genera: Aspergillus, Fusarium, Penicillium and Claviceps.

The chemical structures of mycotoxins produced by these fungi are very diverse, as are the mycotoxicoses they can cause.

The term *mycotoxin* was coined in 1962 after an unexplained die-off of about 100,000 turkeys.

It was then discovered that the mysterious turkey's disease was tied to a feed essentially composed of peanuts contaminated by secondary metabolites of Aspergillus flavus or aflatoxins (Bennett & Klich, 2003).

Mycotoxins are invisible, odourless molecules, and cannot be detected by taste (Binder, 2007).

It is difficult to define mycotoxin in a few words. It is a natural low-molecular-weight molecule; it is a secondary metabolite produced by molds that has adverse effects even at low concentrations on the health of humans, animals, and crops. Those metabolites constitute a toxigenically and chemically heterogeneous class.

Mycotoxins are classified from the a chemical viewpoint into: cyclopeptides, polycetoacids, terpenes, and nitrogenous metabolites, depending on their biological origin and structure (Bhat et al., 2010).

They are mainly produced by the filamentous structure of molds mycelia. They have no biochemical significance for the growth and development of the fungus itself. Over 400 mycotoxins have been isolated and chemically characterized, though research has focused on those forms causing significant harm to humans, animals and crops (Hussein & Brasel, 2001; Zain, 2011). Aflatoxins (AFLs), Ochratoxins A (OTA), trichothecenes as Vomitoxin (DON), Zearelenone (ZEA), Fumonisins B1 and B2 (FUMO B1, FUMO B2), tremorgenic toxins, and ergot alkaloids are the most important mycotoxins if we consider their effects on human health.

It is very important to note that some molds are capable of producing more than one mycotoxin and some mycotoxins are produced by more than one species of mold.

The presence of mycotoxins in cereals, wine, beef, pork and oil seed and other food products has been accepted as natural in many of the EU countries, in the U.S.A, in Canada, Russia, and in most of the Asian Countries (Bhat et al., 2010; Van Egmond & Jonker, 2004).

Mycotoxins are not destroyed by cooking and by normal industrial food processing since they all are heat-stable.

Exposure to mycotoxins may result in a variety of illnesses that fall under the heading of mycotoxicosis, from ingestion or in occupational circumstances from dermal and inhalation exposure (Jarvis & Miller, 2005; Li et al., 2011; Straus, 2011).

Human exposure to mycotoxins may occur at all levels of the food chain: via consumption of plant-derived products contaminated with toxins (cereal grains, coffee, oil seeds, spices, fruit juices, and beverages as wine and beer), or even from carrying-over of mycotoxins and their metabolites (e.g. aflatoxin M1) in milk, meat, and other products of animal origin contaminated because of using feeds with mycotoxins (Bhat et al., 2010; CAST, 2003), or by exposure to air and dust containing toxins (Jarvis, 2002;). In recent times, in actual fact, concerns have been raised about exposures to mycotoxins in indoor environments as a damp houses and buildings (Straus, 2011).

In Ferrante and colleagues study (2007) was carried out a monitoring of wheat samples because it is the main ingredient of bread and pasta, basic aliments, and quantitatively substantial of Mediterranean diet. Wheat samples, from various areas of East Sicily, was analyzed for carcinogenic micotoxins (AFLs, OTA, ZEA). The results show that all samples collected do not contained AFLs whereas OTA and ZEA have been found in the samples to medium concentrations of 0.01 mg/kg and 0.108 mg/kg, respectively. Instead all samples contained OTA and ZEA. So this study confirmed the previous findings of the related studies present in literature.

The main mycotoxins that contaminate food rarely are found in indoor environments.

Indeed, Penicillium and Aspergillus are the main contaminants of both food and damp buildings, though in the latter they produce different mycotoxins.

The genera found in outdoor air, as Aspergillus and Penicillium, are not associated with human or animal toxicosis.

The molds associated with buildings comprise a narrow group of species that grow thanks to the nutrients present in building materials and to the available water (Jarvis & Miller, 2005; Straus, 2011).

A. versicolor, that is often encountered in damp buildings, typically produces *Sterigmatocystin,* a class 2B carcinogen (IARC, 1993; Jarvis & Miller, 2005).

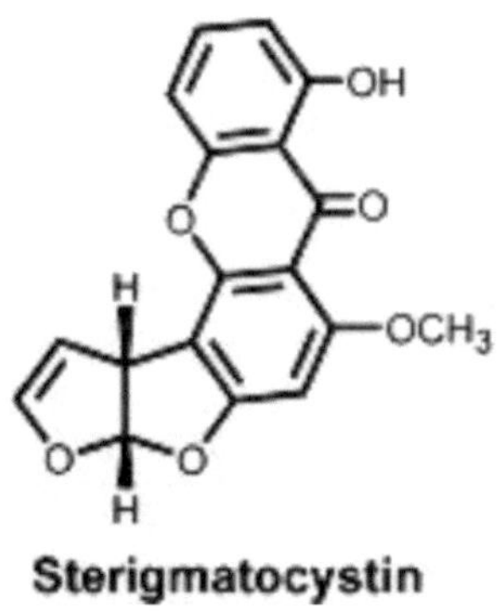

Fig. 2. Molecular formula of Sterigmatocystin.

The most frequent toxigenic fungi in Europe are Aspergillus, Penicillium and Fusarium (Bhat et al., 2010; Creppy, 2002), while the prevalence of specific toxins around the world is as follows: AFLs in Africa and in the Asian continent; AFLs and FUMO in Australia; AFLs, OTA,

ZEA and DON in North America; AFLs , FUMO, OTA, DON and T-2 toxin in South America; ZEA and DON in the Eastern European Countries; OTA, ZEA and DON in the Western European regions (Bhat et al., 2010; Van Egmond & Jonker, 2004; WHO, 2002a). However, with the open global trade these mycotoxins might also be detected in all areas of the world.

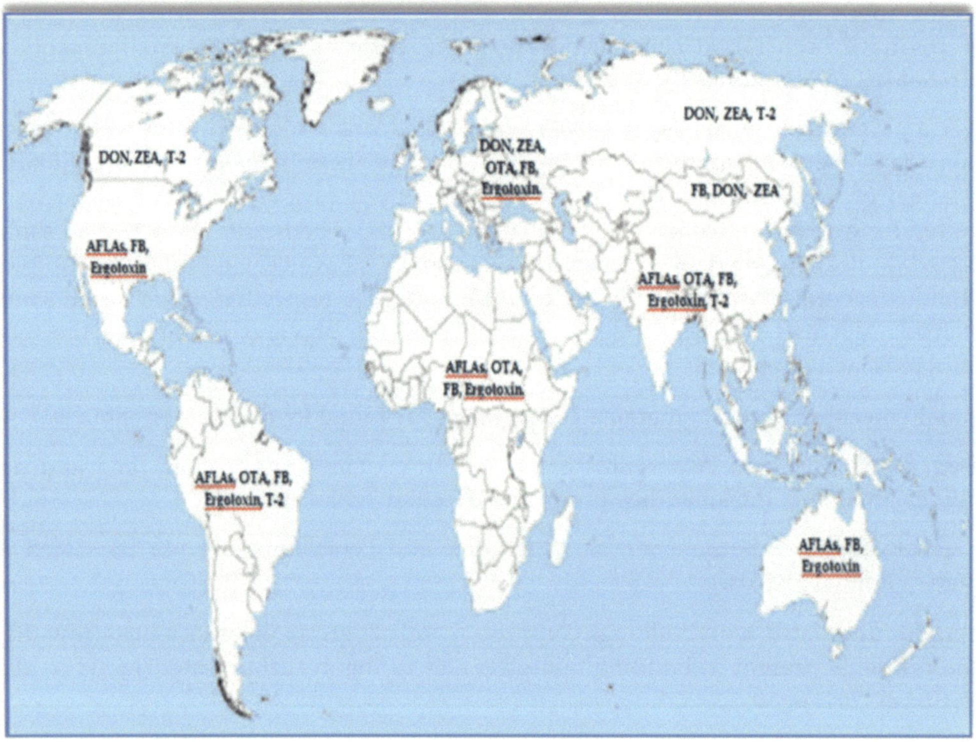

Fig. 3. Distibution of mycotoxins around the world. (AFLAs: Aflatoxins; FB: Fumonisins; OTA: Ochratoxin A; ZEA: Zearalenone; T-2: T-2 toxin).

At this stage, in Europe mycotoxins are controlled, but the regulatory policies still need to be standardized in the various European Countries.

Factors contributing to the presence or production of mycotoxins in foods or feeds include storage, environmental and ecological conditions, but also farming activities, such as drying, handling, packaging and transport, contribute to molds growth and to increase the production of mycotoxins when good practices are not followed (Zain, 2011).

Researchers have found a variety of factors operating interdependently in the production of mycotoxins. Those factors have been categorized as physical, chemical, and biological.

Physical factors include environmental characteristics as temperature, relative humidity, and insect infestation.

Chemical factors include the use of fungicides or fertilizers; biological factors, instead, depend on the interactions between the colonizing toxigenic fungi and the substrate, in fact some plant species are more susceptible to colonization while environmental conditions may increase the vulnerability of others that are more resistant (Zain, 2011).

2. Health effects from dietary exposure to mycotoxins

Concern about mycotoxins is based on well-documented human mycotoxicosis such as ergotism in Europe, alimentary toxic aleukia (ATA) in Russia, acute aflatoxicosis in South and Est Asia, and human primary liver cancer in Africa and South Est Asia.

OTA, instead, is suspected to be a causal factor of Balkan Endemic Nephropathy (BEN) in Yugoslavia and *chronic interstitial nephritis* (CIN) in North Africa.

More epidemics, associated with economic losses and war, have occurred in Russia (1924 and 1944), Ireland (1929), France (1953) and Ethiopia (1978) (Murphy, 2006).

The first episodes of lethal disease in humans caused by ATA have been in Russia, followed by other Countries.

This devastating disease, often fatal, is characterized by necrotizing, hemorrhagic and central nervous system effects and has been identified as a toxic manifestation of grain contamination by mold.

Retrospectively, it has been proven to be caused by; toxins, a metabolite of *Fusarium sporotrichioides*, the most common fungus isolated from contaminated grains incriminated in this russian disease (Richard, 2007; Li et al., 2011).

Still today, especially in developing Countries, mycotoxicoses represent a serious problem, difficult to prevent.

In Africa, many acute diseases are associated with mycotoxins, like aflatoxic hepatitis in Kenya and the vascular ergotism in Ethiopia. From studies carried out on people in Kenya, Mozambique and Swaziland, higher levels of AFLAs were found in food and these were correlated with levels detected in human fluids as urine and blood (Sibanda et al., 1997).

It is hard to define mycotoxins, as well as to classify them. The classification schemes tend to reflect the training of the categorizing person (Zain, 2011).

Mycotoxins cause various and powerful deleterious effects on human health, as some of them are carcinogenic, mutagenic, teratogenic, estrogenic, hemorrhagic, immunotoxic, nefrotoxic, hepatotoxic, dermotoxic and neurotoxic (see Table. 1).

AFLs are important causal factors of liver cancer while FUMO and OTA are suspected to have an important role in the etiology of esophageal cancer and in the famous BEN *(Balkan Endemic Nephrotoxicity)* respectively (Tab. 2.).

The impact of mycotoxins on health depends on various factors, as the fungus species, the daily intake of the mycotoxins consumed and their concentration, the toxicity of the compound, their mechanisms of action, the body weight of the individual, the presence of other synergic or protective elements present in the food, the metabolism and defense mechanisms of the host (Hussein & Brasel, 2001; Stayn, 1995).

Their toxic effects, however, are mostly proven in experimental models.

The inaccuracy of extrapolation of results for humans is an important point for research; it may be explained by the lack of adequate food consumption data, by the gap of knowledge about health risks associated with the actual proposed limits and by the big possibility of synergism or additive toxicity with other mycotoxins present in the same food (Creppy, 2002).

Genera	Mycotoxins	Biological effect
Aspergillus		
	Aflatoxin B1	Carcinogenic, mutagenic, immunotoxic, hepatotoxic
	Aflatoxin G1	Carcinogenic, mutagenic, immunotoxic, hepatotoxic
	Aflatoxin M1	Carcinogenic, mutagenic, immunotoxic, hepatotoxic
	Ochratoxin A	Carcinogenic, teratogenic, immunotoxic, nefrotoxic
	Sterigmatocystin	Carcinogenic , mutagenic, teratogenic
	Cyclopiazonic acid	Mutagenic, neurotoxic
Penicillium		
	Patulin	Genotoxic, mutagenic
	Ochratoxin A	Carcinogenic, teratogenic, immunotoxic, nefrotoxic,
	Citrinin	Nefrotoxic
	Penitrem A	Neurotoxic
	Cyclopiazonic acid	Mutagenic, neurotoxic
Fusarium		
	Vomitoxin	Hemorrhagic, dermotoxic
	Nivalenol	Hemorrhagic, dermotoxic
	Zearalenone	Estrogenic, dermotoxic
	T-2 toxin	Hemorrhagic, dermotoxic
	Diacetoxyscirpenol	Hemorrhagic
	Fumonisins	Carcinogenic
	Moniliformin	Hemorrhagic
	Tenuazonic acid	Hemorrhagic
Alternaria		
	Alternariol	Foetotoxic, teratogenic, hemorrhagic
	Alternariol methyl ether	Foetotoxic, teratogenic, hemorrhagic
Claviceps		
	Ergot alkaloids	Neurotoxic

Table 1. Some mycotoxins and their biological effects on human health.

Mycotoxins	Desease
Aflatoxins	Aflatoxicosis
	Hepatocarcinogenicity
	Encephalophaty
	Reye's sindrome
Ochratoxin A	Balcan Endemic Nephropathy (BEN)
	Kidney tumors
Sterigmatocystin	Pulmonary tumours
	Hepatocarcinogenicity
	Urinary tract tumors
	Kidney tumors
Fumonisins	Esophageal cancer
	Hepatocarcinogenicity
	Pulmonary edema
	Leukoencephalomalacia
	Hepatotoxicity
	Nephrotoxicity
Zearalenone	Cervical cancer

Table 2. List of mycotoxins and relative pathologies.

2.1 Carcinogenic mycotoxins and their mechanisms of action

2.1.1 Aflatoxins

The main aflatoxins include aflatoxins B1, B2, G1 and G2 (see Fig. 4) produced by *Aspergillus flavus* and *A. parasiticus* that contaminate plants and plant products.

Among all aflatoxins, the Aflatoxin B1 (AFB1) is the most potent hepatocarcinogenic substance known; recently, after a thorough risk evaluation, it has been proven to be also genotoxic (Van Egmond & Jonker, 2004; Zain, 2011).

In 1993, the WHO-International Agency for Research on Cancer (WHO-IARC, 1993 a,b) evaluated the carcinogenic potential of Aflatoxins and they were classified as carcinogenic for humans (Group 1). In particular, studies have shown that AFB1 may act in synergy with hepatitis B virus in human hepatocellular carcinoma.

For this type of carcinogen, it is generally felt that there is no threshold dose below which no tumor formation would occur. In other words, only a zero level of exposure will result in no risk.

Aflatoxins are known to bind DNA and induce mutagenic and carcinogenic effects in rats. Especially the AFB1 is bioactivated from its original form to a mutagenic and carcinogenic metabolite (Hussein & Brasel, 2001).

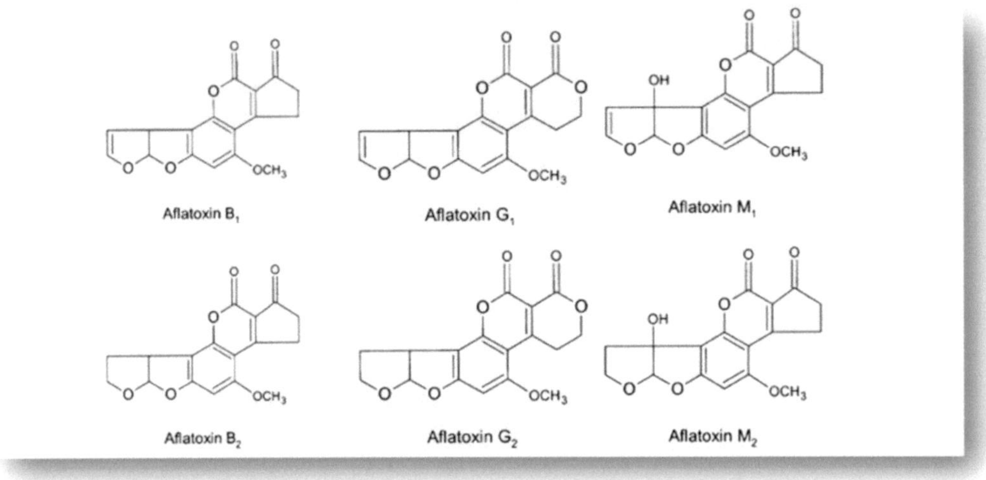

Fig. 4. Molecular formula of Aflatoxins and their metabolites.

Aflatoxins have been found also in tissues of children suffering from Kwashiorkor and Reye's syndrome, that has led to the hypothesis that they could also be causal factors for these diseases.

Reye's syndrome, in particular, is characterized by liver and kidney enlargement and cerebral edema (Hussein & Brasel, 2001).

Aflatoxins M1 (AFM1) and M2 (AFM2) are the hydroxylated metabolites of aflatoxin B1 (AFB1) and B2 (AFB2) respectively and may be found in milk products obtained from livestock that have ingested contaminated feed.

Aflatoxins can be present in cows milk, pork meat or chicken eggs if those animals were exposed to aflatoxins in their feed. The main sources of aflatoxins in feeds are peanuts, meal maize and cottonseed meal (Creppy, 2002; McLean & Dutton, 1995; Richard, 2007).

The concentration of AFB1 in feed can be strongly reduced thanks to good manufacturing and storage practices. If those preventive measures fail, however, AFB1 can be reduced in feed by blending (or diluition) or by physical or chemical treatments. Physical treatments include heat, microwaves, gamma-rays, X-rays and ultra-violet light (Creppy, 2002).

About 0.3–6.2% of AFB1 from animal feed is transformed into AFM1 in milk. The toxicity of AFM1 is about one order of magnitude less than that of AFB1 (Creppy, 2002; Van Egmond & Jonker, 2004 ; Voss et al., 2002).

AFM1 is a possible carcinogenic to humans.

In literature are not yet known specific exposure biomarkers for aflatoxins.

The AFM1 intake from milk is calculated to be 6.8 ng/person per day for the European diet, 3.5 ng/person per day for the Latin American diet, 12 ng/person per day for three son per day for the Middle Eastern diet and 0.1 ng/person per day for the African diet (Creppy, 2002).

Aflatoxins have been regulated with limits in many Countries of the world; for more detailed information see section 6.

2.1.2 Ochratoxin A

OTA or (N-[(3R)-(5-chloro-8-hydroxy-3-methyl-1-oxo-7-isochromanyl)-carbonyl]-l-phenylalanin) (Fig. 5), is a mycotoxin produced by several strains of Aspergillus and Penicillium species, and it is generally associated with a variety of products, such as cereals, coffee beans, cocoa beans, and dried fruit (Abrunhosa et al., 2010; Aragua´s et al., 2005; Juan et. al., 2008).

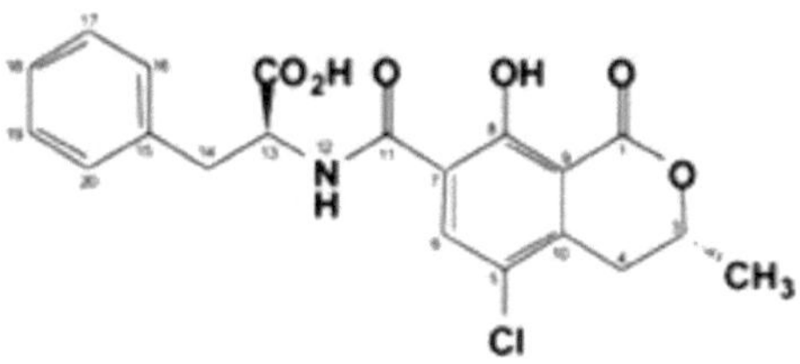

Fig. 5. Chemical structure of OTA.

OTA consists of a dihydroisocoumarin subunit, which is linked to phenylalanine through a peptide bond.

OTA toxicity has been intensively studied (Mally & Dekant, 2009; Abrunhosa et al., 2010); the kidney is the target of OTA toxicity in all animal species exposed to this mycotoxin.

Dietary human exposure to OTA is been suspected to be involved in BEN, a progressive kidney disease associated with an increased risk for the development of urothelial cancers, that occur in some rural areas of Bosnia, Bulgaria, Croatia, Romania, and Serbia.

OTA has a very high affinity to plasma proteins, as 99.9% of the circulating OTA is bound to plasma proteins.

OTA is poorly metabolized and slowly excreted with plasma half-life of 230 hrs in humans (Mally & Dekant, 2009).

Inappropriate farm management practices have been associated with higher OTA amounts. It is also known that meat may contain OTA through secondary contamination and carry-over (Pfohl-Leszkowicz & Manderville, 2007).

Studies have not completely identified so far the mechanism nor the extent of the carcinogenic potential of OTA in humans; therefore, OTA is classified by IARC as possible carcinogen (Group 2B) (Abrunhosa et al., 2010).

The provisional tolerable weekly intake (PTWI) for OTA established by the Joint FAO/WHO Expert Committee on Food Additives and Contaminants is 100 ng/kg bw/week (Juan et al., 2008; Kabak, 2009; Pfohl-Leszkowicz & Manderville 2007).

Some scientist have shown that the DNA lesions (on dG exclusively) induced by OTA in vivo exposure were no longer repaired in case of repeated exposure; these lesions could then be proposed as a marker of exposure in populations at risk (Creppy, 2002; Abrunhosa et al., 2010).

Prevention of growth of *A. ochraceus* consists in application of standard practices as rapidly and thoroughly drying the grains and also fumigation, aeration and cooling, sealed storage and controlled atmosphere.

An important preventive factor for correlated pathologies is the diet rich in antioxidants, vitamins, amino acids and aspartame. In fact positive and protective effects of aspartame in kidney and brain have been reported. Actually aspartame is used for prevention of OTA genotoxicity in kidneys (Creppy, 2002).

Several studies are available on OTA-induced nephrotoxicty and renal tumor formation.

The OTA mechanisms of action are divided into direct (covalent DNA adduction) and indirect (oxidative DNA damage) (Pfohl-Leszkowicz & Manderville, 2007; Mally & Dekant, 2009; Reddy & Bhoola, 2010).

Oxidative DNA damage induced by direct oxidation of DNA constituents or through oxidative stress has been implicated in renal tumor formation and it represents the most accepted theory in current literature (Mally & Dekant, 2009; Abrunhosa et al., 2010).

However, currently the OTA carcinogenicity pathway is unknown because it has not yet been observed sperimentally.

Several pathways of kidney tumorigenicity by ochratoxin have been proposed by scientists:

- DNA-adduct formation
- Oxidative stress
- Cell proliferation
- Modulation of apoptosis
- Alteration of gene expression

(Kamp et al., 2005; Kuan et al., 2008; Mally & Dekant, 2009 ; Reddy & Bhoola, 2010).

EFSA has recently established a tolerable weekly intake (TWI) of 120 ng/kg of body weight for OTA. While the exposure of the general population in Europe is below this TWI, additional data regarding OTA-exposure of infants and children are considered necessary to account for their specific dietary preferences and needs (EFSA, 2006; Kabak, 2009; Mally & Dekant, 2009).

2.1.3 Sterigmatocystin

Sterigmatocystin, or (3a*R*,12c*S*)-8-hydroxy-6-methoxy-3a,12c-dihydro-7*H*-furo[3',2':4,5]furo[2,3-*c*]xanthen-7-one (Fig. 6) is a toxic metabolite closely related to the aflatoxins structure and consists of a xanthone nucleus attached to a bifuran structure. The IARC have included the sterigmatocystin in group 2B, which means it is a likely carcinogenic to humans.

Sterigmatocystin is generally produced by the fungi *Aspergillus nidulans* and *A. versicolor* (Veršilovskis & De Saeger, 2010).

It has been found in mouldy grain, green coffee beans and cheese although current information on its occurrence in foods is again incomplete and poor.

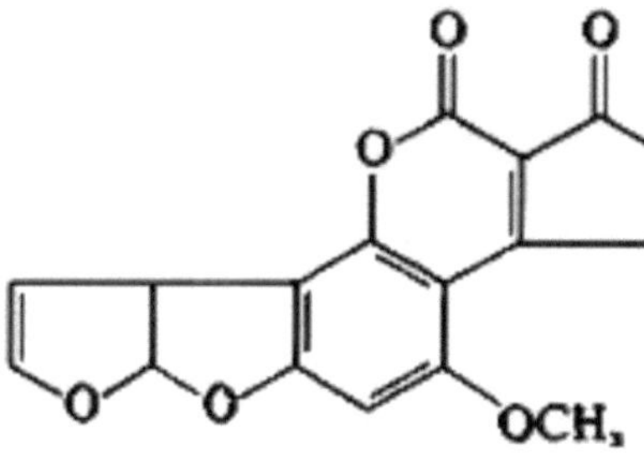

Fig. 6. Chemical structure of Sterigmatocystin

It appears to occur much less frequently than the aflatoxins perhaps because the analytical methods for its determination have not been as sensitive, therefore it is possible that small concentrations of Sterigmatocystin in food commodities may at times not have been detected. Sterigmatocystin is considered a potent carcinogen, mutagen and teratogen toxin. A number of closely related compounds such as o-methyl Sterigmatocystin are known and some may occur naturally.

Effects of chronic exposure that have been reported include induction of hepatomas in rats, pulmonary tumours in mice, renal lesions and alterations in the liver and kidneys of African monkeys. Rats fed with 5-10 mg/kg of sterigmatocystin for two years showed a 90% incidence of liver tumours.

The acute toxicity, carcinogenicity and metabolism of Sterigmatocystin have been compared to those of aflatoxin and several other hepatotoxic mycotoxins.

Contamination by Sterigmatocystin usually occurs in wheat, maize, animal feed, hard cheese, pecan nuts and green coffee beans but also in cereals, grain products, fruits and marmalade, dried meat products and grapefruit juice.

Relatively high levels of sterigmatocystin have been formed in bread, cured ham and salami after inoculation with *A. versicolor*. No country has legislation for sterigmatocystin; however, it is important to emphasize that the natural occurrence of this mycotoxin appears to be infrequent, though only a limited number of surveys have been carried out (Noda et al., 1981; Stich & Laishes, 2006; Veršilovskis & De Saeger, 2010).

2.1.4 Fumonisin

Fusarium verticillioides, F. moniliforme and *F. proliferatum* are the fungi that produce significant quantities of fumonisins (Fig. 7 and Fig. 8). Today at least 15 related fumonisin compounds have been identified but the fumonisin B1 or diester of propane-1,2,3-tricarboxylic acid (FB1) (Fig. 6) and fumonisin B2 (FB2) (Fig. 7) are the predominant forms. The fumonisins are highly water-soluble because they lack an aromatic structure.

Fumonisins occur in maize and corn and infrequently in foodstuffs such as sorghum, asparagus, rice, beer and beans (Creppy, 2002; Murphy, 2006; Zain, 2011).

The IARC has classified Fumonisins as possible human carcinogens (Class 2B). Consumption of fumonisin has been associated with elevated human esophageal cancer incidence in various parts of Africa, China, Central America, and among the black population in Charleston, South Carolina, USA (Hussein & Brasel, 2001; Murphy et al., 2006).

FB1 is responsible for leukoencephalomalacia (necrotic lesions in the brain) in horses and pulmonary edema in swine. Hepatotoxicity and nephrotoxicity effects have also been reported in connection with chronic dietary exposure to fumonisin. Fumonisins are also a real risk factor in neural tube and related teratogenic defects because they reduce folate uptake (Zain, 2011).

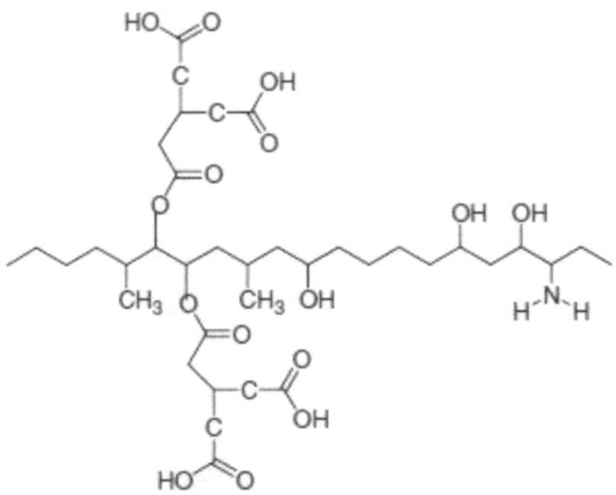

Fig. 7. Chemical structure of FMB1

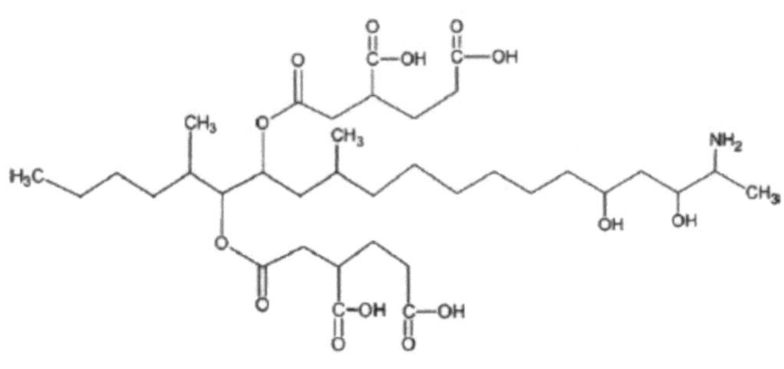

Fig. 8. Chemical structure of FMB2.

Fumonisins are known to disrupt sphingolipid synthesis and concentrations; thus, the altered plasma sphingosine/sphinganine ratios is an important biomarker of fumonisin dietary exposure (Murphy et al., 2006).

Many biochemical pathways have been postulated to explain the induction of illnesses by fumonisins. Several hypotheses are proposed and all are related to disruption of lipid metabolism as the initial step.

Some researchers have proposed that the first mechanism involves disruption of sphingolipid metabolism through inhibition of ceramide synthase. Glycerophospholipid metabolism is also affected (Voss et al., 2002).

A second theory proposes a biochemical mechanism that involves the fatty acid disruption, Glycerophospholipid metabolism, the relative induction of oxidative stress but also an incorrect modulation of gene expression.

Fumonisin has been unequivocally shown to be genotoxic, in fact DNA adducts of fumonisin B1 have been found.

A provisional maximum of tolerable daily intake (PMTDI) for FB1, FB2 and FB3, individually or in combination, is fixed at 2 µg/kg of body weight per day on the basis of the NOEL of 0.2 mg/kg of body weight per day and a safety factor of 100 (Creppy, 2002).

2.1.5 Zearalenone

Zearalenone (Fig. 9) is a mycotoxin produced by *F. graminearum* and other *Fusarium* molds as *F. culmorum, F. cerealis, F. equiseti,* and *F. semitectum,* using corn, wheat, barley, oats and sorghum as substrates. *Fusarium* infects cereals in the field. Toxin production occurs before harvesting, but also post harvest if the crop is not handled and dried properly (see section 6).

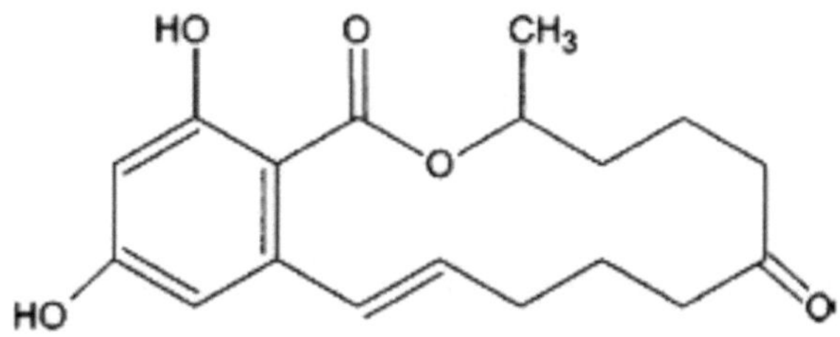

Fig. 9. Chemical structure of ZEA

Among the human population, children are the most affected due to consumption of ZEA-contaminated foods (mainly cereals and cereal-based food products) (Massart & Saggese, 2010). This toxin is worldwide distributed and can contaminate most of the cereals like barley, maize, oats, sorghum, millet, rice, soybeans but also wheat and bread. ZEA has been implicated in several incidents of early puberty, as it is suspected to be the causative agent in an epidemic of early puberty changes in young children in Puerto Rico.

ZEA is a non-steroidal compound that exhibits oestrogen-like activity in some farm animals (e.g. cattle, sheep and pigs) and it is a 6-(10-hydroxy-6-oxo-trans-1-undecenyl)-b-resorcylic acid l-lactone.

Altogether ZEA may have a species-dependent carcinogenic effect possibly secondary to the hormonal effect (Massart & Saggese, 2010); however, no data about formation of DNA-adducts in humans are actually available.

ZEA and some of its metabolites have been shown to competitively bind to oestrogen receptors (α-zearalenol and β-zearalenol); all of them have been included by IARC in Group 3, as not classifiable as carcinogens to humans.

Human adenocarcinomas and endometrial hyperplasia found in ZEA contaminated women are still under investigation (Bhat et al., 2010; Codex Alimentarius Commission, 2000; Creppy, 2002; Massart & Saggese, 2010; Zain, 2011).

No international homogeneous maximum limit exists in foodstuff for ZEA. Eight countries of the World have specific regulations for ZEA ranging from 30 to 1000 µg/kg.

The JECFA has established a provisional maximum tolerable daily intake for ZEA to be 0.5 µg/kg of body weight (JECFA, 2000).

The Canadian daily intake of ZEA from maize and maize-based cereals has been estimated to be 0.005 - 0.087 µg/kg b.w. for 12 - 19 year-old males, the highest consumption group. An additional intake from popcorn was estimated to be 0.001 - 0.023 µg/kg b.w.

3. Combined toxic effects of mycotoxins

It has been known for many years that several products derived from plants contaminated by fungi during plant growth or during harvest and storage of the food item, can contain more types of mycotoxins; as a consequence, food intake results in a simultaneous exposure to a mix of mycotoxins; for example, often citrinin and ochratoxin A are found together (see Table 3).

There are several combinations of mycotoxins that frequently occur as verified by specific monitoring programs. These combinations are summarized in Table 3.

Mycotoxins	References
OTA and Citrinin	Pohland et al., 1992; Vrabcheva et al., 2000; Pfohl-Leszkowicz et al. 2007
OTA and ZEA	Halabi et al. 1998
AFB1 , FB1 and ZEA	Oliveira et al., 2006
OTA and AFB1	Sedmikova et al., 2001
FB1 and Moniliformin	Gutema et al., 2000
DON, NIV, T2, HT-2	Eskola et al., 2001
DON, NIV, T2, HT-2, ZEA	Tanaka et al., 2010

Table 3. Combinations of mycotoxins in food.

When mycotoxins are of similar structure and of the same species or of the same family, it is likely to expect similar mechanism of action, therefore mycotoxins are likely to exert additive effects. However, there are relatively poor information on the interaction between mycotoxins that occur at the same time and the consequences for animal and human health.

The available data in literature show that adequate studies to establish antagonistic, additive or synergistic effects after combined exposure to mycotoxins are rare and some of them are difficult to interpret.

The few studies conducted on the mycotoxins co-presence have shown that combined exposure to several mycotoxins generally results in an additive toxic effect with a few exceptions. The synergic capacity is relatively small for NIV, DON, T-2, ZEA and FB1.

The interaction between NIV and T-2 has been seen as synergistic because the effect of T-2 is potentiated in the presence of high levels of NIV (Berthiller et al., 2009; Bouslimi et al., 2008; Speijers & Speijers, 2004; Tammer et al., 2007).

It would be proper for future research to try to understand how mycotoxins can interact and thus interfere between them.

4. Ghost mycotoxins

Mycotoxins may also occur in conjugated forms such as:

- soluble or masked mycotoxins
- mycotoxins incorporated into/associated with/attached or bound to macromolecules.

Conjugated mycotoxins can be produced after metabolization by living plants, fungi and mammals, after food processing or because of some cooking methods.

It has been shown that wheat enzymatically produces deoxynivalenol 3-glucoside (D3G) from DON to defend itself from the very same toxin attack.

During storage, on the contrary, the plant product generally has a low metabolic activity and its enzymatic protections may not be as active.

Mycotoxins can be altered by subsequent food processing and most frequently through conjugation. The reliable analytical methods, measurement standards and occurrence and toxicity for this forms of mycotoxins are still lacking.

So, the risk assessment from exposure of consumers to mycotoxins should also take into account the presence of those forms (Berthiller et al., 2009; Bouslimi et al., 2008; Tammer et al., 2007).

4.1 Fungal conjugates

Some mycotoxin conjugates can be excreted directly by fungi, although examples are rare. This is the case of the well known 3-acetyl deoxynivalenol (3ADON) and 15-acetyl deoxynivalenol (15ADON), that can be found in cereals contaminated by *Fusarium*. Both substances are biosynthetic precursors of DON.

Some strains of *F. sambucinum* and *F. sporotrichoides* produce compounds such as 4-propionyl HT-2 toxin, 8-nhexanoyl neosolaniol, 8-butyryl neosolaniol, 8-isobuturyl neosolaniol, and 8-pentenoyl neosolaniol in hydroponics culture.

Zearalenone 4-sulfate (Z4S) was found to be a natural *Fusarium* metabolite.

Similarly, *Rhizopus arrhizus* is capable of catalysing sulfation of ZEA to Z4S. (Berthiller et al., 2009; Tammer et al., 2007).

4.2 Plant conjugates

Plants protect themselves from xenobiotic compounds like mycotoxins by converting them into more polar metabolites.

It remains unclear, however, whether glycosylated mycotoxins are less toxic than the storage forms or they are part of the mechanism of the plant self-protection.

In wheat and maize cell suspension cultures OTA is transformed into ochratoxin α and methylester-ochratoxin A (two isomers of hydroxyochratoxin A) as well as into their glucosides and methyl esters.

Fumonisin conjugates were long believed to occur only after food processing but recently it has been shown that bound fumonisins could also be found in unprocessed maize.

The exact chemical nature of these naturally occurring hidden forms is still unknown. In particular, it has to be understood whether conjugates are formed by the plant from non covalent interactions, e.g. with starch or proteins.

4.3 Food-processing conjugates

Food processing, especially heating and fermentation, can potentially alter some mycotoxins. D3G in fact was detected in malt and beer made from barley naturally contaminated with Fusarium, but also DON conjugates with higher masses as diglucosides and triglucosides have been detected in beer. Generally, very little is known regarding bound mycotoxins.

Depending on the type of linkage to proteins, starch, pectins, hemicellulose, cellulose and lignin, it is possible that at least some of the bound mycotoxins could become bioavailable again in the digestive tract of humans and animals.

Conjugation does not occur only during food processing; an excessive heat can also alter mycotoxins structure considerably; in fact, although mycotoxins are very stable, thermal degradation products of NIV and DON have been found in food and feed.

Fumonisins conjugates with sugars, amino acids and proteins are known to occur in food and feed. Heating FB1 with reducing sugars can yield N-(carboxymethyl) FB1, even in corn products.

Protected lysine and cysteine methyl esters react with FB1 demonstrating that free groups as thiol or amino groups of proteins are likely to react with the mycotoxins. Furthermore, it has been proven that thermal food processing influences the chemical structure and toxicity of fumonisins (Berthiller et al., 2009; Bouslimi et al., 2008; Speijers & Speijers, 2004; Tammer et al., 2007).

4.4 Mammalian conjugates

Conjugates that arise from mammalian metabolization unlikely have a role in food or feedstuffs and are therefore not regarded as masked mycotoxins.

Mycotoxins are conjugated by humans and animals during metabolization in the liver and are excreted in urine. Serum albumin adducts of AFB1 can be formed by Patulin that has been shown to react with cellular nucleophiles such as proteins or glutathione. This is the most probable pathway of detoxification in man and animals after dietary exposure to patulin-contaminated apples.

The ability to form glutathione and cysteine conjugates has also been shown for ochratoxin A. The most common mycotoxin conjugation products in mammals are glucuronides, as found for the *Fusarium* mycotoxins DON and ZEA. Besides the unchanged mycotoxins, both deoxynivalenol glucuronides and zearalenone glucuronide were detected in the urine of exposed animals.

Some DON and ZEA sulfates are formed and excreted by animals too. These conjugates might be used as biomarkers; by doing so, also inhalation of mycotoxins (e.g. by grain workers or from indoor moulds) and the consumption of all bioavailable forms of mycotoxins (including masked mycotoxins) might be monitored (Berthiller et al., 2009; Bouslimi et al., 2008; Speijers & Speijers, 2004; Tammer et al., 2007).

5. Mycotoxins control strategies, a possible form of prevention

Good agricultural practices (GAPs), good manufacturing practices (GMPs), HACCP (Hazard Analytical Critical Control Point), biological control measures and transgenic approaches, are actually the only realistic and possible form of primary prevention for mycotoxins flowering.

A control program for mycotoxins from the field to the table should include the HACCP approach, thus requiring an understanding of the interactions of the toxigenic fungi with crop plants, of the production and harvest methods for crops, of the production of livestock using grains and processed feeds, a thorough knowledge including diagnostic capabilities for mycotoxicoses, the development of new practices of foods processing for human consumption including storage and delivery (Jard et al., 2011).

A good protocol for mycotoxins checking is necessary to manage all control points and finally for being able to ensure to the consumer a food supply free from mycotoxins (Binder, 2007 ; Richard, 2007; Abrunhosa et al., 2010).

The results of HACCP show that the products obtained have an elevated hygienic quality, thus lowering the risk of contamination. The dried pasta, for example, is one of the foods most commonly consumed by Italians and Italy is leading the world ranking for the consumption of pasta. Also, pasta is conquering more and more important positions in the dietary habits of various peoples. The study of Ferrante and colleagues (2009) was to assess the presence of ZEA and OTA with the aim of identifying the consumer's risk.

The results of this study have showed OTA and Zea concentrations below the limit of methods in all types of dried pasta tested, also have showed that the HACCP system adopted by Italian food industries are adequate for preserve the food quality. This study moreover have showed in particular that the products for celiac consumers and the products made with whole wheat flour have an elevated hygienic quality.

The efficient storage systems can be also a good practice for reduction of contamination by mycotoxins.

One of the conservation techniques for food is the lyophilization. Ferrante and colleagues in 2006 carried out the study for verify presence of : tri-5 gene, ZEA, NIV and DON, in the primary products used for the preparation of lyophilized foodstuffs and in their final products (prontocrepes and prontocone).

The study have showed that the Tri-5 gene are always present in prontocrepes and always absent in prontocone products. With the air treatment a reduction of DON and NIV in both products has been obtained. The nitrogen treatment has had a single influence on the DON and in both final products, in which has had a reduction to 50 %. While, the NIV with the same treatment has reached the lowest percentage of reduction in both final products. The treatments affect relatively on the contamination of processed-foods that, therefore, in this case was due on the first quality of the primary products.

Populations residing in developed Countries are usually considered to be less exposed to mycotoxins than those in developing Countries; this might be attributed to various factors:

- execution and practice of modern food handling/preservation technology
- successful governmental regulation and commercial control over food quality and safety.

However, even monitoring and exercising of good agricultural and manufacturing practices (GAP and GMP) along with an effective HACCP approach might not completely avoid or eliminate mycotoxins in the food chain (Bhat, 2010; Jard et al., 2011; Zain, 2011).

5.1 Biological control

Various biocontrol strategies are possible for reducing the levels of mycotoxins in the crops, such as development of atoxigenic bio-control fungi that can out-compete their closely related, toxigenic strains in field environments.

It has been reported the existence of non-toxigenic strains of *A. flavus* and *A. parasiticus* that can reduce the post-harvest aflatoxin contamination by 95.9%.

The competitive use of biological agents such as *F. verticillioides* strains was observed to suppress the growth of fumonisin-producing fungi.

Control of fumonisins producing fungi by endophytic bacteria has also been reported and competitive exclusion was thought to be the mechanism involved.

It has also been reported that Pichia anomala, Pichia kluyveri and Hanseniaspora uvarum can inhibit in vitro OTA.

Furthermore, fungal strains of Trichoderma have been demonstrated to control pathogenic molds through mechanisms such as competition for nutrients and space, fungistasis, rhizosphere modification, mycoparasitism, biofertilization and the stimulation of plant-defense mechanisms (Bhat, 2010; Jard et al., 2011; Zain, 2011).

5.2 Chemical control

Appropriate use of pesticides during the production period could help in minimizing fungal infections or insect infestation of crops and consequently mycotoxins contamination; therefore, Fumonisins contamination could be reduced by application of fungicides that have been used for controlling Fusarium, such as prochloraz, propiconazole, epoxyconazole, tebuconazole, cyproconazole and azoxystrobin.

On the other hand, fungicides such as itraconazole and amphotericin B have been shown to effectively control the aflatoxin-producing Aspergillus species. However, use of fungicides is been discouraged because of economic, environment and severe food safety issues (Bhat, 2010; Jard et al., 2011; Zain, 2011).

5.3 Decontamination

Decontamination of food and feed from mycotoxins could be achieved through chemoprotection or enterosorption.

Chemoprotection from aflatoxins has been demonstrated with the use of a number of chemical compounds like oltipraz and chlorophylin or through dietary interventions based on broccoli sprouts and green tea that increase animal's detoxification processes or prevent the production of epoxide, that is known to cause chromosomal anomalies.

However, this intervention might not be sustainable in the long-term because it is expensive and shows some side effects.

Entersorption is based on the discovery of certain clay minerals, such as Novasil, that can selectively adsorb mycotoxins enough to prevent their absorption from the gastrointestinal tract .

There are different adsorption agents but their efficacy in preventing mycotoxicosis varies. Calcium montorillonites have proven to be the most highly selective and effective of enterosorbents. However, with enterosorption, there is a risk that non-specific adsorption agents may prevent uptake of micronutrients from the food (Bhat, 2010; Jard et al., 2011; Zain, 2011).

5.4 Breeding for resistance

Breeding for resistance is the most promising and encouraged long-term strategy for control of mycotoxins contamination in Africa. Sources of resistance to *A. flavus* and *Fusarium spp.* have been identified, particularly *F. verticillioides.*

Zain (2011) states that "Prototypes of genetically engineered crops have been developed that

a. contain genes for resistance to the phytotoxic effects of certain trichothecenes, thus helping reducing fungal virulence or
b. contain genes encoding fungal growth inhibitors for reducing fungal infection in the USA".

To devise effective strategies to control fungal infections and minimize mycotoxins production in host plants, a good knowledge of genetic variability and plants population structure is necessary (Kazan et. al., 2011; Jard et al., 2011; Zain, 2011).

6. Regulation of mycotoxins in foods and feeds

A series of studies on mycotoxins in food and feed have been carried out around the world in order to improve policy making.

Regulations relating to mycotoxins have been established in many Countries to protect consumers from the harmful effects of these compounds. In 2003 about 100 Countries (covering approximately 85% of the world's inhabitants) had already specific regulations or detailed guidelines on mycotoxins in food. Regulations concerned AFB1, AFB2, AFG1, AFG2 and AFM1, trichothecenes (Vomitoxin, diacetoxyscirpenol, T-2 toxin and HT-2 toxin), FB1, FB2, and FB3, agaric acid, ergot alkaloids, OTA, patulin, phomopsins and ZEA, leaving out sterigmatocystin.

Harmonized EU limits now exist for 40 mycotoxin–food combinations. The direct or indirect influence of European organizations and programs on the EU mycotoxins regulatory developments was significant.

The current maximum limits are more and more based on scientific evidence from authoritative agencies such as FAO/WHO, Joint Expert Committee on Food Additives of the United Nations (JECFA) and the European Food Safety Authority (EFSA) (Van Egmond & Jonker, 2004).

The FDA has action levels for aflatoxins but the European Community levels are more restrictive (Creppy, 2002; Mally & Dekant, 2009).

Efforts have continued internationally to establish better guidelines to control mycotoxins. FAO, for example, has worked with developing Countries (African and East-Asian Countries) to mitigate mycotoxins contamination in foods and feeds.

Many Countries have regulatory or guideline limits for OTA in foods but in the majority of cases OTA content limits have been established only for cereals and cereal products (see Tab. 5).

There are still some discussions in those organizations regarding the limit that should be established for OTA in some cereal-derived foods, in fact in some Countries there is no limit or it is not harmonized with the international level (see Tab. 5) (Araguás et al., 2005).

Limit of AFB1 on ppb (µg/kg)	Number of countries	Limit of AFB1, B2,G1,G2 on ppb (µg/kg)	Number of countries
25	1	35	2
20	3	30	3
15	2	20	17
10	5	15	8
5	21	10	8
2	29	5	3
1	1	4	29
20	3	3	1
		1	3
		0	2

Table 4. Worlwide limits for AFB1 and sum of AFB1, B2, G1, G2 in food.

Many Countries, even if industrialized, such as USA and Canada, still today lack of legal limit for AFB1, showing how the problem is unfortunately underestimated.

Furthermore, looking at Table 5, it is also evident that still today in many Countries of the world there are no limits for OTA, ZEA and Fumonisins, and that worldwide regulations for sterigmatocystin are completely lacking.

Several Countries, such as Bahamas, Bolivia, Burkina Faso, Cameroon, Ecuador, Ethiopia, Iraq, Myanmar, Nicaragua, Pakistan, Panama, Qatar, Trinitad and Tobago, Uganda, United Arab Emirates, Yemen, Zambia and Zimbawe, until 2003, hadn't yet established any regulations or limits for any mycotoxins, that means that the carcinogenic risk to which local populations are subjected is high.

Myctoxin	Country	Maximum limit (ppb)	Food
AFB1	EU*	2	Food, peanuts, shell fruits, dried fruits, cereals
		5	Unprocessed maize , spices and tea
		8	Unprocessed peanuts
		0.1	Cereal and other complementary foods for infants and small children
		0.1	Dietary foods for special medical purposes (specifically for infants)
		2	Maize, cereals
	Algeria	10	Peanuts, nuts, cereals.
	Armenia	5	All foods
	China	20	Maize and maize products, peanut and peanut products, peanut oil, irradiated peanut
		10	Rice, irradiated rice, edible vegetable oil
		5	Soya bean sauce, grain paste, vinegar, other grains, beans, fermented foods, fermented bean products, starch products, fermented wine, red rice, butter cake, pastry biscuit and bread
	Croatia	5	Cereals, beans, peanuts, coffee, tea
		30	Spices
	Cuba	5	Cereals, peanuts, cocoa mass
	Egypt	5	Peanuts and cereals
	Honduras	1	Maize
		10	Corn
	Iran	10	Barley
		5	Pistachio nuts, peanuts, walnuts, other nuts, edible seeds, dates, dried grapes (raisins and sultanas), figs and all dried fruits, maize, rice, wheat, legumes
		0.5	Baby food based on cereals with milk
		1	Baby food based on cereals without milk
	Israel	5	Nuts, peanuts, maize flour, figs and their products and other foods
	Japan	10	All foods
	Jordan	15	Almonds, cereals, maize, peanuts, pistachio nuts, pine nuts, rice
	Korea Rep.	10	Grains, soy-bean, peanuts, nuts, wheat and the products made from these by simple processing
	Malawi	5	Peanuts export
	Moldova Rep.	5	Cereals, legumes, flour, cocoa, nuts, coffee, sunflower, tea
	Morocco	10	Wheat bran and all foods
		5	Vegetable oils, cereals, wheat meal

Myctoxin	Country	Maximum limit (ppb)	Food
		1	Peanuts, pistachio nuts, almonds, vegetable oils in pasta, children foods
	Nepal	20	Cereals
	Nigeria	20	Foodstuffs
	Oman	10	Foodstuffs
	Russia	5	All foods
	Senegal	50	Peanut products
		300	Peanut products (feedstuff ingredients)
	South Africa	5	All foodstuffs
	Switzerland	1	All foods
	Tanzania Rep.	5	Cereals, oil seeds
	Tunisia	2	All foods
Σ (B1, B2, G1, G2)	EU*	4	Peanuts , dried fruits, cereals and related products intended for direct human consumption
		15	Unprocessed peanuts
		10	Unprocessed shell fruits, dried fruits
		10	Maize unprocessed, spices and thea.
	Algeria	20	Peanuts, nuts, cereals.
	Australia§	15	Peanuts, tree nuts
	Barbados	20	All foods
	Bosnia & Herzegovina	1&	Cereals
		5	Beans
	Canada	15	Nuts and nut products
	Chile	5	All foods
	Colombia	10	All foods
		20	Maize
	Costa Rica	35	Maize
	Croatia	3	Cocoa beans, almonds, flours, hazelnuts, walnuts
	Cuba	5	All foods
	Dominican Rep.	0&	Maize(products), groundnut, soya, tomato(products)
		20	Imported maize
	Egypt	10	Peanuts , cereals
		20	Corn
	Guatemala	20	Maize, kidney beans, rice, sorghum, groundnuts, and groundnut butter
	Honduras	1°	All foods
		0.01&	Baby food
	India	30	All foods
	Indonesia	20	Peanuts, coco nuts, spices, traditional drugs, erbs
	Iran	15	Pistachio nuts, peanuts, walnuts, other nuts, edible seeds, dates, dried grapes (raisins and sultanas), figs and all dried fruits,wheat

Myctoxin	Country	Maximum limit (ppb)	Food
		10	Legumes
		50	Barley
		30	Maize, rice
	Israel	15	Nuts, peanuts, maize flour, figs and their products and other foods
	Jamaica	20	Food, grains
	Jordan	30	Almonds, cereals, maize, peanuts, pistachio nuts, pine nuts, rice
	Kenya	20	Peanuts, vegetable oils
	Kuwait	0.2	Milk and milk products(except dried milk)
		0.05	Infant and children food
	Macedonia	1[&]	Wheat, maize, rice and cereals
		5[&]	Beans
	Malaysia	35	All foods
	MERCOSUR[+]	20	Peanuts, maize and products thereof
	Mexico	20	Cereals and products
		12	Corn flour for tortillas
	Mozambique	10	Peanut, maize, peanut butter, peanut milk
	Philippines	20	Nut products
	Salvador El	20	All foods
	Saudi Arabia	0.05	Infant and children food
	Singapore	5	Corn, nuts, and cereal products
	South Africa	10	All foodstuffs
	Switzerland	5°	All foods
	Taiwan	15	Peanut, corn, maize
		10	Rice, sorghum, legumes, nuts, wheat and barley, oats, edible oils and fats
	Tanzania Rep.	10	Cereals, oil seeds
	Thailand	20	All foods
	USA	20	All foods
	Venezuela	20	Corn, corn flour, peanuts, peanut butter
	Vietnam	10	Foodstuffs
AFM1	EU*	0.025	Newborn and baby food
		0.05	Milk and derivates
	Armenia	0.5	Milk
	Barbados	0.5	Milk
	Chile	0.05	Milk
	China	0.5	Milk and milk products
	Croatia	0.5	Milk and milk products
	Honduras	0.05	Milk and milk products
		0.02	Baby food
		0.25	Cheese
	India	30	Milk and milk products

Myctoxin	Country	Maximum limit (ppb)	Food
	Indonesia	5	Milk, cheese
	Iran	0.02	Baby food based on cereals with milk
		0.5	Milk powder
		0.01	Milk powder for babies
		0.2	Cheese
		0.02	Butter, gee
	Israel	0.05	Milk and milk products
	Korea Rep.	0.5	Milk and milk products
	MERCOSUR+	0.5	Milk
		5	Milk powder
	Moldova Rep.	0.5	Milk, cottage cheese, butter
	Morocco	0.05	Milk and milk products
		0.03	Milk (product) for infants under 3 years
		0.5	Milk powder
		0.3	Milk powder for infants under 3 years
	Russia	0.5	Milk and milk products
	Singapore	0.5	Milk, cheese
	South Africa	0.05	Milk
	Switzerland	0.02	Newborn and baby food
		0.05	Milk and milk products
		0.250	Cheese
	Taiwan	0.5	Milk
		5	Milk powder
	USA	0.5	Milk
	Venezuela	0.5	Milk
		5	Milk powder
OTA	EU*	5	Unprocessed cereals
		3	Cereals and processed cereal-based food intended for direct human consumption
		10	Dried grapes (raisins and sultanas)
		5	Roasted coffee beans and ground roasted coffee, with the exception of instant coffee
		10	Instant coffee
		2	Wine (red, white and rosé) and other wine and / or other drinks based on grape must. Grape juice, based ingredients of grape juice
		2	Cocoa and chocolate powder
		0.5	Cereal and other complementary foods for infants and dietary foods for special medical purposes (specifically for infants)
		0.5	Chocolate and its derivatives
		0.2	Beer
		1	Pork and derivatives
	Cuba	5	Coffee, cereals
	Indonesia	Not detectable	Coffee

Myctoxin	Country	Maximum limit (ppb)	Food
	Iran	50	Barley, maize
		20	Legumes
		10	Dates, dried grapes (raisins and sultanas), figs and all dried fruits
		5	Rice, wheat
		1	Baby food based on cereals without milk
	Israel	50	Cereals, cereal products and other foods
	Morocco	30	Cereals
	Singapore	2.5	Cereal, raw coffee beans and roasted coffee beans
	Sudan	15	Wheat
	Switzerland	2	Cereals
FB1+ FB2	EU*	4000	Unprocessed maize
		1000	Maize intended for direct human consumption, maize-based foods for direct human consumption
		800	Maize-based breakfast cereals and maize-based snacks
		200	Processed maize-based foods and baby foods for infants and young children
	Cuba	1000	Maize, rice
	Switzerland	1000	Maize
	USA	2000	Unprocessed maize
ZEA	EU*	20	Processed maize-based foods for infants and young children
		100	Unprocessed cereals other than maize
		350	Unprocessed maize
		400	Refined maize oil
		75	Cereals intended for direct human consumption, cereal flour, bran and germ.
		50	Bread pastries, biscuits, cereal snacks and breakfast cereals, excluding maize-snacks and maize-based breakfast cereals
		100	Maize intended for direct human consumption, maize-based snacks and maize-based breakfast cereals
		100	Maize intended for direct human consumption
	Armenia	1000	All foods
	Chile	200	All foods
	Indonesia	Not detectable	Maize
	Iran	400	Barley

Myctoxin	Country	Maximum limit (ppb)	Food
		200	Maize, rice, wheat
	Moldova Rep.	1000	Wheat , barley, maize and their flour
	Morocco	200	Cereals and vegetable oils
	Russia	1000	Cereals and vegetable oils

Eu*= 27 countries (Austria, Bulgaria, Cyprus, Czech. Rep., Denmark, Estonia, Finland, France, Germany, Greece, Hungary, Ireland, Italy, Latvia, Lithuania, Luxembourg, Malta, The Netherland, Poland, Portugal, Romania, Slovakia, Slovenia, Spain, Sweden, Great Britain). Norway, Iceland and Liechtenstein to follow the limits of the European Union (harmonized standards).
° = Σ (B2, G1 and G2).
&= Σ (B1+G1).
§= All Australian regulations were harmonized with New Zealand.
+= MERCOSUR member states: Argentina, Brazil, Paraguay and Uruguay.

Table 5. Worldwide maximum limit of carcinogenic mycotoxins for food.

7. Conclusions and future research

Besides the demonstrated effects of mycotoxins on humans and animals, some important aspects of their toxicology and possible control mechanism are still unknown and unexplored. The occurrence of mycotoxins in the food chain is therefore an unavoidable and serious problem that the world is facing not without efforts nor difficulties.

The toxic effects of mycotoxins (on liver and kidney, hematopoietic toxicity, immune system toxicity, reproductive system toxicity, foetal toxicity and teratogenicity, and moreover carcinogenicity) are mostly known in experimental models but the extrapolation for humans is often inaccurate.

The inaccuracy of extrapolation for humans may be explained by the lack of adequate food consumption data and/or lack of knowledge about relative health risks associated with specifically proposed limits and finally by the gap of knowledge on the possibility of synergism with other mycotoxins present in the same food products.

Wide gaps still exist on the toxicological effects of feeding animals with mycotoxin-contaminated feeds.

Further research also needs to be focused on epidemiology of toxic effects, especially in humans.

Development of new genetically modified plants by the application of genetic engineering that might be resistant to fungal invasion might also prove today to be a good option for preventing growth of toxigenic fungi, though they leave open many question marks in any case.

Development of methods for simple, rapid and economic analysis chemical contaminants throughout the food chain. The researchers Ferrante and Oliveri Conti have carried out the development of a method for simultaneous determination of 13 mycotoxins and some their metabolites in LC-MS tandem TQD in serum and urine of humans (Article awaiting acceptance by journal) after enzyme treatment of samples.

Even though research papers, reviews, monographs, and government reports are available on the contamination of food and feed by fungal toxins, nonetheless most of the information are restricted to only one type of mycotoxin (Bhat et al., 2010), and they do not take into account ghost mycotoxins.

Much still needs to be done, both at governmental and scientific level, in order to reach higher standards of protection for consumers. It is important to harmonize as soon as possible the maximum limits for food taken from Country to Country due to global trade, that increases the risks due to mycotoxins ingestion in the population of the importing Country.

8. Acknowledgments

The authors gratefully acknowledge the contribution of Dr. Pasquale Di Mattia in terms of comments, medical English and constructive suggestions provided for improving the manuscript.

9. References

Abrunhosa L.,. Paterson R.R.M., Venâncio A., (2010). *Biodegradation of Ochratoxin A for Food and Feed Decontamination*. Toxins, 2:1078-1099.

Aragua´s, C., Gonza´lez-Pen˜as, E., Lo´pez de Cerain, A (2005). Study on ochratoxin A in cereal-derived products from Spain. Food Chemistry, 92 : 459–464.

Bhat, R., Rai, R.V., Karim, A.A. (2010). *Mycotoxins in Food and Feed: Present Status and Future Concerns.* Comprehensive Reviews in Food Science and Food Safety, Vol.9, 57-81.

Berthiller, F., Schuhmacher, R., Adam, G., Krska, R. (2009). *Formation, determination and significance of masked and other conjugated mycotoxins.* Anal Bioanal Chem., 395: 1243-1252.

Binder, E.M. (2007). *Managing the risk of mycotoxins in modern feed production.* Animal Feed Science and Technology, 133: 149–166.

Bouslimi, A., Bouaziz, C., Ayed-Boussema, I., Hassen, W., Bacha, H. (2008). *Individual and combinated effects of ochratoxin A and citrinin on viability and DNA fragmentation in cultured Vero cells and on chromosome aberrations in mice bone marrow cells.* Toxicology, 251:1-7.

Bünger, J., Westphal, G., Mönnich, A., Hinnendahl, B., Hallier, E., Müller M., (2004). *Cytotoxicity of occupationally and environmentally relevant mycotoxins*. Toxicology, 202: 199–211.

CAST, (2003). *Mycotoxins: Risks in Plant, Animal and Human Systems.* Report No. 139. Council for Agricultural Science and Technology, Ames, Iowa, USA.

Creppy, E.E. (2002). *Update of survey, regulation and toxic effects of mycotoxins in Europe.* Toxicology Letters 127, pp 19–28.

Codex Alimentarius Commission (2000), FAO-WHO, Joint FAO/WHO Food Standards Programme, Codex Committee on Food Additives and Contaminants, *Position Paper on Zearalenone.* pp1-5.

EFSA, 2006. *Opinion of the CONTAM Panel related to ochratoxin A in food.* EFSA. EFSA-Q-2005-154.

Eskola, M., Parikka, P., Rizzo, A., (2001). *Trichothecenes, ochratoxin A and zearalenone contamination and Fusarium infection in Finnish cereal samples in 1998*. Food Addit. Contam., 18: 707–718.

European Commission (2006). *The Rapid Alert System for Food and Feed (RASFF) Annual Report 2005*. Health and Consumer Protection Directorate-General, Office for Official Publications of the European Communities, Luxembourg.

Ferrante, M., Agodi, A., Fallico, R., Fiore, M., Barchitta, M., Brundo, M.V., Carpinteri, G., Di Mattia, P., Galata,' R., Longhitano, F., Maugeri, M., Oliveri Conti, G., Sciacca, S. (2006). *Contamination Evaluation Of Lyophilizated Processed-Foods.* Epidemiology, Vol.17 - Issue 6 - p S298, ISEE/ISEA 2006- Conference Abstracts Supplement .

Ferrante, M., Fiore, M., Oliveri Conti, G., Sinatra, M.L., Ledda, C., Castronovo, M., Fallico, R., Sciacca, S. (2007). *AFLs, OTA, and ZEA in Wheat Samples Come From East Sicily*.Epidemiology. 18(5):S118.

Ferrante, M., Oliveri Conti, G., Ledda, C., Sciacca, G.E., Fiore, M., Sinatra, M.A., Cunsolo, M., Fallico, R., Sciacca, S. (2009) *Ota and Zea in dried pasta on the Italian market.* 17th Annual EUPHA Meeting, European Journal of Public Health, Vol. 19, Supplement 1, pag 145.

Gutema, T., Munimbazi, C., Bullerman, L.B., 2000. *Occurrence of fumonisins and moniliformin in corn and corn-based food products of U.S. origin.* J. Food Protect. 63: 732-737.

Kabak, B. (2009). *Ochratoxin A in cereal-derived products in Turkey: Occurrence and exposure assessment.* Food and Chemical Toxicology, 47: 348–352.

Kamp, H.G., Eisenbrand, G., Janzowski, C., Kiossev, J., Latendresse, J.R., Schlatter, J., Turesky, R.J. (2005). *Ochratoxin A induces oxidative DNA damage in liver and kidney after oral dosing to rats.* Mol. Nutr. Food Res., 49: 1160 – 1167.

Kuan, M.M., Cavin, C., Delatour ,T., Schilter, B. (2008). *Ochratoxin A carcinogenicity involves a complex network of epigenetic mechanisms.* Toxicon, 52: 195–202.

Kazan K., Gardiner D.M., Manners J.M. (2011). *On the trail of a cereal killer: recent advances in Fusarium graminearum pathogenomics and host resistance.* Mol Plant Pathol., doi: 10.1111/j.1364-3703.2011.00762.x. [Epub ahead of print].

Halabi, K.S., Natour, R.M., Tamini, S.O., (1998). *Individual and combined effects of chronic ochratoxin A and zearalenone mycotoxins on rat liver and kidney*. Arab Gulf J. Scient. Res.,16, 379–392.

Hussein, S. H., Brasel, J.M. (2001). *Toxicity, metabolism, and impact of mycotoxins on humans and animals* Toxicology, 167: 101–134.

IARC (1993). *Some naturally occurring substances: food items and constituents, heterocyclic amines, and mycotoxins.* IARC Monogr, 56: 489–520.

Jard, G., Liboz, T., Mathieu, F., Guyonvarc'h, A., Lebrihi, A. (2011). *Review of mycotoxin reduction in food and feed: from prevention in the field to detoxification by adsorption or transformation.* Food Addit Contam Part A Chem Anal Control Expo Risk Assess, 28(11):1590-609.

Jarvis, B.B., 2002. *Chemistry and toxicology of molds isolated from water-damaged buildings. Mycotoxins and food safety*. Adv. Exp. Med. Biol. 504, 43–52.

Jarvis, B.B., Miller, J.D. (2005). *Mycotoxins as harmful indoor air contaminants.* Appl Microbiol Biotechnol, 66: 367–372.

JECFA. Joint Expert Committee on Food Additives. 2000. Joint FAO/WHO Expert Committee on Food Additives, 53rd report. *Safety evaluation of certain food additives.* WHO food additives series 44.

Juan, C., Pena, A., Lino, C., Moltó, J.C., Mañes, J., Juan, C., Pena, A., Lino, C., Moltó, J.C., Mañes J. (2008). *Levels of ochratoxin A in wheat and maize bread from the central zone of Portugal.* International Journal of Food Microbiology 127: 284–289.

Li, Y., Wang, Z., Beier, R.C., Shen, J., De Smet, D., De Saeger, S., Zhang, S. (2011). *T-2 toxin, a trichothecene mycotoxin: review of toxicity, metabolism, and analytical methods.* J Agric Food Chem., 59(8):3441-53.

Massart, F., Saggese, G.(2010).*Oestrogenic mycotoxin exposures and precocious pubertal development.* Int J Androl., 33(2):369-76.

Mally, A., Dekant, W. (2009). *Mycotoxins and the kidney: Modes of action for renal tumor formation by ochratoxin A in rodents.* Mol. Nutr. Food Res., 53: 467–478.

McLean, M., Dutton, M.F. (1995). *Cellular interaction and metabolism of aflatoxin: an update.* Pharmac. Ther., Vol. 65, pp 163-192.

Murphy, P. A., Hendrich, S., Landgren, C., Bryant, C. M. (2006). *Food Mycotoxins: An Update.* Journal Of Food Science, Vol. 71, Nr. 5, pp 51-65.

Noda, K., Umeda, M. , Ueno, Y. (1981). *Cytotoxic and mutagenic effects of sterigmatocystin on cultured Chinese hamster cells.* Carcinogenesis, 2(10): 945-949.

Oliveira, G.R., Ribeiro, J.M., Fraga, M.E., Cavaglieri, L.R., Direito,G.M., Keller, K.M., Dalcero, A.M., Rosa, C.A.(2006). *Mycobiota in poultry feeds and natural occurrence of aflatoxins, fumonisins and zearalenone in the Rio de Janeiro State, Brazil* . Mycopathologia, Vol. 162, N.5, pp 355-362.

Pfohl-Leszkowicz, A., Manderville, R A. (2007). *Ochratoxin A: An overview on toxicity and carcinogenicity in animals and humans.* Mol. Nutr. Food Res., 51: 61–99.

Pfohl-Leszkowicz, A., Tozlovanu, M., Manderville, R., Peraica, M., Castegnaro, M., Stefanovic, V. (2007). *New molecular and field evidences for the implication of mycotoxins but not aristolochic acid in human nephropathy and urinary tract tumor.* Molecular Nutrition & Food Research, Vol. 51, Issue 9, pages 1131–1146.

Pohland, A.E., Nesheim, S., Friedman, L., 1992. *Ochratoxin A: A review.* Pure Appl. Chem. 64, 1029–1046.

Reddy L., Bhoola K. (2010). *Ochratoxins-Food Contaminants: Impact on Human Health.*Toxins, 2: 771-779.

Richard, J.L. (2007). *Some major mycotoxins and their mycotoxicoses – An overview.* International Journal of Food Microbiology, 119: 3–10.

Riley, R.T., (1998). *Mechanistic interactions of mycotoxins: theoretical consideration.* In: Sinha, K.K., Bhatanagar, D. (Eds.), Mycotoxins in Agriculture and Food Safety. Marcel Dekker, Inc, Basel, New York, pp. 227–254.

Rouzer, C.A. (2011). *Bypassing A Toxic DNA Adduct: A Look Into The Enzyme Active Site.* VICB Communications. Vanderbilt Institute of Chemical Biology. Vanderbilt University.

Sedmikova, M., Reisnerora, H., Dufkova, Z., Burta, I., Jilek, F. 2001. Potential hazard of simultaneous occurrence of aflatoxin B1 and ochratoxin A. Vet. Med., 46: 169-174.

Sibanda, L., Marovatsanga, L.T., Pestka, J.J. (1997). *Review of mycotoxin work in sub-Saharan Africa.* Food Control, Vol. 8, No.1, pp 21-29.

Speijers, G.J.A., Speijers, M.H.M. (2004). *Combined toxic effects of mycotoxins.* Toxicology Letters, 153: 91–98.

Steyn, P.S. (1995). *Mycotoxins, general view, chemistry and structure.* Toxicology Letters, 82/83: 843–851.

Stich, H.F., Laishes, B. A. (2006). *The response of Xeroderma pigmentosum cells and controls to the activated mycotoxins, aflatoxins and sterigmatocystin.* International Journal of Cancer, vol.16, issue 2.

Straus, D.C.(2011). *The possible role of fungal contamination in sick building syndrome*. Front Biosci (Elite Ed), 3:562-80.

Tammer, B., Lehmann, I., Nieber, K., Altenburger, R., (2007). *Combined effects of mycotoxin mixtures on human T cell function*. Toxicol Lett, 170: 124-133.

Tanaka, H., Sugita-Konishi, Y., Takino, M., Tanaka, T., Toriba, A., Hayakawa, K. (2010). *A survey of the occurence of Fusarium mycotoxins in biscuits in Japan by using LC/MS*. Journal of Health Science., 56(2): 188-194.

Van Egmond , H.P., Jonker, M.A. (2004) . *Worlwide regulations for mycotoxins in food and feed in 2003*. The Food and Agriculture Organization of the United Nations (FAO).

Veršilovskis, A., De Saeger, S. (2010). *Sterigmatocystin: Occurrence in foodstuffs and analytical methods – An overview*. Molecular Nutrition & Food Research., Vol. 54, Issue 1, pp136–147.

Voss, K.A., Howard, P.C., Riley, R.T., Sharma, R.P., Bucci, T.J., Lorentzen, R J. (2002) *Carcinogenicity and mechanism of action of fumonisin B1: a mycotoxins produced by Fusarium moniliforme (=F. verticillioides)*. Cancer Detection and Prevention, 26: 1–9.

Vrabcheva, T., Usleber, E., Dietrich, R., Märtlbauer, E., (2000). *Co-occurrence of ochratoxin A and citrinin in cereals from Bulgarian villages with a history of Balkan endemic nepropathy*. J. Agric. Food Chem., 48, 2483–2488.

WHO. 2002a. *WHO Global Strategy for Food Safety: safer food for better health*. Food Safety Programme 2002. World Health Organization (WHO), Geneva, Switzerland.

Zain, M.E., (2011). *Impact of mycotoxins on humans and animals*. Journal of Saudi Chemical Society, 15: 129–144.

8

Food Borne Carcinogens: A Dead End?

Rosa Busquets Santacana
University of Brighton,
United Kingdom

1. Introduction

One of the major challenges in biomedicine is to find strategies to prevent cancer. It is among the top 10 causes of death in middle and high income countries (WHO, 2004) and accounts for a major economic expenditure; for instance, £5.86 billion were spend on cancer care in 2009-2010 in the UK, which is 5.6% of the UK´s total annual health spending (Sullivan et al., 2011). The pathogenesis of this condition involves a series of complex and interwoven mechanisms ranging from genetic to environmental and/or behavioral factors. Some of the causes and risk factors of cancer are smoking, infection/inflamation, dietary factors, sunlight exposure, and pollution (Sugimura, 2002). Radiofrequency electromagnetic fields have also been recently classified as "possibly carcinogenic" by the World Health Organization's International Agency for Research on Cancer (IARC) (IARC, 2011). This chapter is going to focus mainly on diet as a risk factor for cancer.

Diet can play an important role in the onset of cancer since apparent harmless meals, to which we are exposed daily, can bring mutagens in close proximity to our DNA, certainly a bad combination. The formation of the "cooking mutagens" takes place in the framework of the Maillard reaction when thermally treating food. These mutagens are products of the reaction of common food components such as aminoacids, fatty acids or creatine and have to be metabolically activated to acquire the potential to alter DNA. For instance, melanoidins, the polymers that give the brownish colour when cooking (Arnoldi et al., 1997; Tehrani et al., 2002), are other products of the Maillard reaction with which we are more familiar.

Study in cooking mutagens was pioneered at Lund University, in 1939, where E.M.P Widmark reported that organic solvent extracts from grilled horse meat caused tumours in mice mammary glands when they were repeatedly applied to mouse skin (Widmark, 1939). Some years later, Druckrey and Preussman (Druckrey et al., 1962) reported the presence of carcinogenic N-nitrosamines in tobacco smoke, which were identified in food in the 1990s (Drabik-Markiewicz et al, 2011; Tricker et al., 1991). The presence of polycyclic aromatic hydrocarbons was also found on the crust of well-done charcoal-grilled steaks by Lijinsky and Shubick. These compounds were formed from the pyrolysis of fat drippings into flames and the adherence of this pyrolysate to the surface of food (Chung, 2011; Lijinsky & Shubick, 1964). Not long after, a revolutionary assay to quantify mutagenic activity was developed by Ames et al. (1975) based on Salmonella typhimurium strains (Ames et al., 1975). This assay helped Sugimura and co-workers to find high mutagenic activity in particles of smoke produced by cooking proteinaceous foodstuffs and immediately afterwards in charred parts of broiled fish and meat (Nagao et al., 1977). Mutagenic activity was also detected in meat prepared under domestic conditions (Commoner et al., 1978). These findings initiated research into heterocyclic amines (HCAs) and since then several series of mutagenic HCAs have been identified. Some potential and new HCAs have been recently reported in thermally treated food (Busquets et al., 2007, 2008; Turesky et al., 2007). HCAs result from the reaction of natural components present in protein rich food at normal cooking conditions. In 2005, the U.S. National Toxicology Program listed four HCAs as reasonably anticipated human carcinogens, status that has been mantained in the latest report (RoC, 2011). Earlier, in 1993, the IARC already listed one HCA as probable human carcinogen (group 2A) and eight HCAs as possible human carcinogens (group 2B) and recommended a decrease in their intake (IARC, 1993). Furan, mainly found in coffee, baby food, beer and canned sauces and soups, was also classified as possibly carcinogenic to humans (Group 2B) (IARC, 1995). This compound is formed from three major routes beginning with sugars, ascorbic acid or unsaturated fatty acids (Al Taki et. al, 2011; Maga, 1979). For a review, see Crews and Castle (Crews & Castle, 2007). Recently, acrylamide, listed within the group 2A (IARC, 1994) and formed from the reaction between asparagine and glucose (Mottram et al., 2002; Tareke et al., 2002;) has also been found in carbohydrate-rich foods. The major exposure to acrylamide mainly appears to come from the consumption of French fries, crisps, biscuits or cereals (Bermudo et al., 2006; Tareke et al., 2002). At present, additional naturally occurring substances such as 5-(hydroxymethyl)-2-furfual (HMF) and related compounds, which are formed from hexoses in acidic media, are being evaluated for their potential human genotoxicity. In particular, high levels of HMF have been quantified in honeys, caramel products, plum-derived products, coffee and balsamic vinegars (Glatt & Sommer, 2006; Teixidó et al., 2006). Some examples of relatively abundant cooking mutagens among the types listed above, are the nitrosamine NMDA (N-nitrosodimethylamine); the polycyclic aromatic hydrocarbon BPA (benzo[a]pyrene); the heterocyclic aromatic amine PhIP (2-amino-1-methyl-6-phenylimidazo[4,5-*b*]pyridine); HMF; furan and acrylamide, shown in Fig. 1.

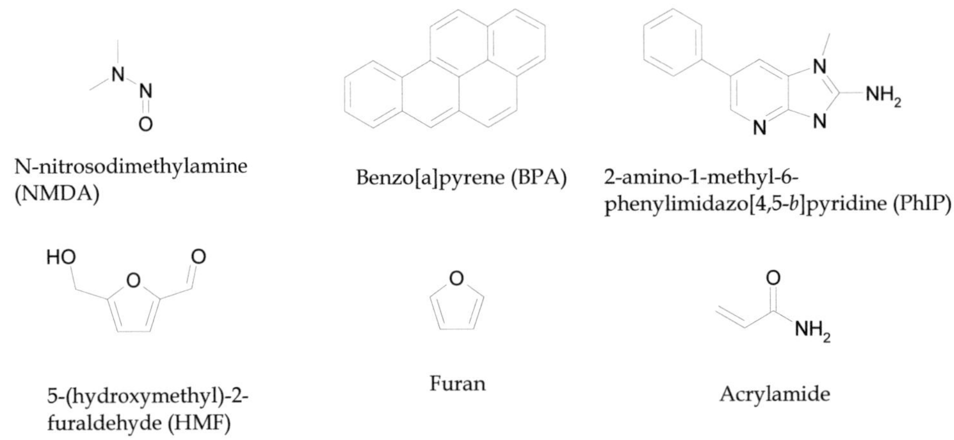

Fig. 1. Examples of food borne mutagens.

When somebody is informed about the generation of potential harmful compounds in common food items, whom asks who or what is responsible for that exposure. The answer to that is our eating preferences and habits, as it will be explained later in this book chapter. Some may recall previous information they had about it "I heard that the charred part of food is not healthy". This is a good start, because it means that research has been disseminated and people are aware to some extent of the lack of safety in burnt food. However the information received is partly innacurate as potential hazardous compounds can also be present in the non overcooked parts of the food. For instance, Fig. 2 shows chicken cooked using different methods and the corresponding concentration of mutagenic HCAs analysed in these food items. It can be seen that non charred meat can contain relatively high levels of cooking mutagens, HCAs in this case. Besides, very different levels of HCAs can be found in an item presenting similar degree of doneness and browning that has been processed using different cooking methods.

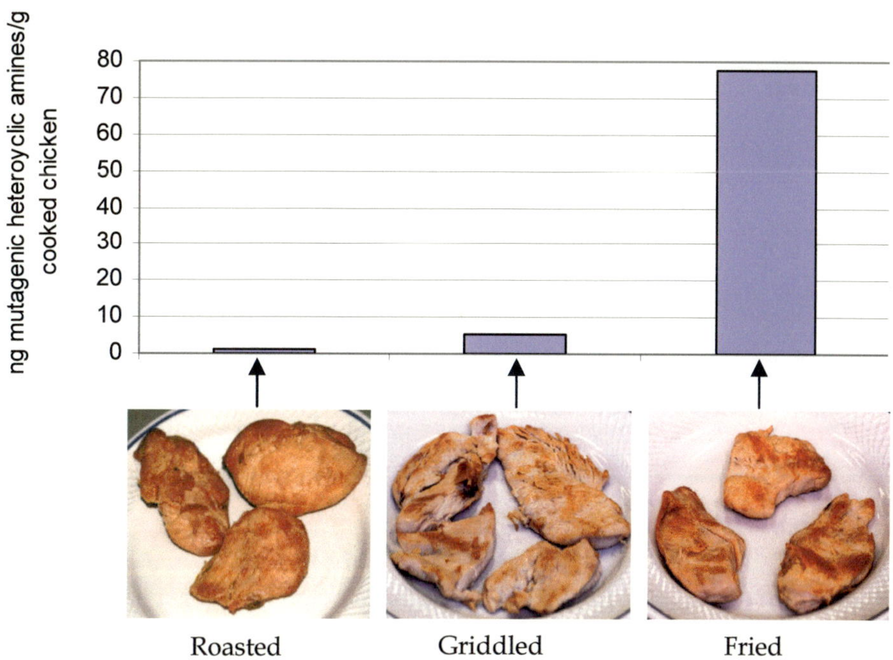

Fig. 2. Level of mutagenic HCAs in chicken cooked in different ways. Each bar corresponds to the concentration of HCAs quantified in the respective item displayed. The cooking and analysis conditions have been reported elsewhere (Busquets et al., 2004, 2008).

Finally, despite the effort of scientists to study food borne mutagens, human behaviour is complex and, in some occasions, the public reacts saying "I like barbecued meat and I love crisps and there is no way I will I stop eating them". In summary, if in the best case people have been warned on the certain risks associated to some food items and they will not make an effort to reduce the exposure, who would care about them; are food borne carcinogens a dead end?

2. Exposure to food borne carcinogens. Heterocyclic amines (HCAs), a case study

The formation of HCAs results from the reaction of hexoses, creatine/creatinine and amino acids (Jägerstad et al, 1983a, 1983b; Murkovic et al., 1999, 2004) and is highly affected by the chemical and physical parameters during the cooking process as well as the composition of the raw food. It is important to understand the effect of such parameters on exposure to HCAs, as an example of food borne mutagens, to understand, to some extent, the absence of legislation, and subsequently the low interest of the companies to monitor or reduce the level of HCAs in food items. The proposed route for the formation of HCAs (quinolines and quinoxalines) is shown in Fig 3 and the proposed mechanism for the formation of pyridinic HCAs is given in Fig. 4.

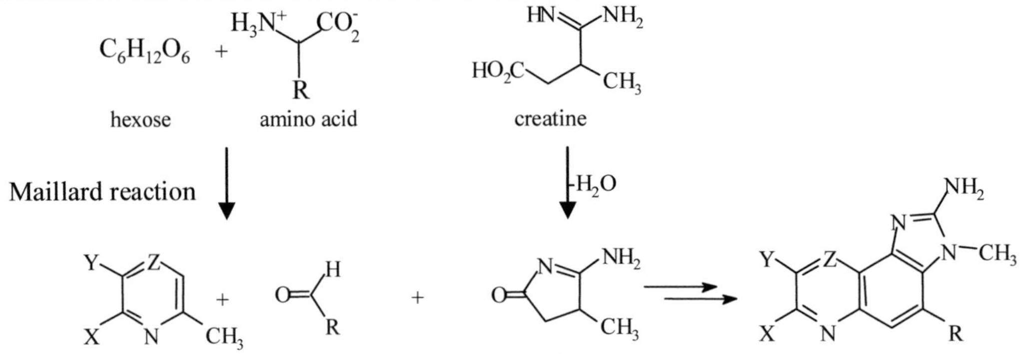

	X	Y	Z	R
IQ:	H	H	CH	H
MeIQ:	H	H	CH	CH_3
MeIQx:	H	CH_3	N	H
7,8-DiMeIQx:	CH_3	CH_3	N	H
4,8-DiMeIQx:	H	CH_3	N	CH_3

Fig. 3. Proposed pathway for the formation of quinoline (IQ, MeIQ) and quinoxale type (MeIQx, 4,8-DiMeIQx and 7,8-DiMeIQx) of HCAs. Adapted from Jägerstad et al. (Jägerstad et al., 1983b).

A study using precursors of PhIP (structure shown in Fig. 1) labelled with 13C was key to clarify the reaction mechanism involved in the formation of this amine, which is the most abundant mutagenic HCA in cooked meat and fish. Phenylalanine labelled with ^{13}C at three non-aromatic positions (C-1, C-2 and C-3) (see Fig. 4) provided important information. When labelling the carbon atom of the carboxylic acid of phenylalanine (C-1), there was no incorporation of ^{13}C, probably due to fast decarboxylation. When labelling the C-2 of the amino acid, two different signals were detected in ^{13}C-NMR (C-5 and C-7 in PhIP); and when labelling at C-3, just one position of PhIP incorporated the ^{13}C (C-3 in PhIP). From these experiments, Murkovic et al. proposed the mechanism of formation of PhIP that is reproduced in Figure 4 (Murkovic et al., 1999). C-1 of phenylacetaldeyde (2), i.e. Strecker degradation product of phenylalanine (1), undergoes aldol condensation with creatine (3) to form (A), which suffers dehydration to form (B). A and B intermediates were isolated from model systems and from heated meat in Dr. Murkovic's research group (Zöchling et al., 2002). Experiments with ^{15}N-labelled phenylalanine, carried out to identify the origin of the nitrogen forming the pyridine moiety of PhIP, revealed that this amino acid was not the only source of this atom, and that creatine or even free ammonia could also provide it.

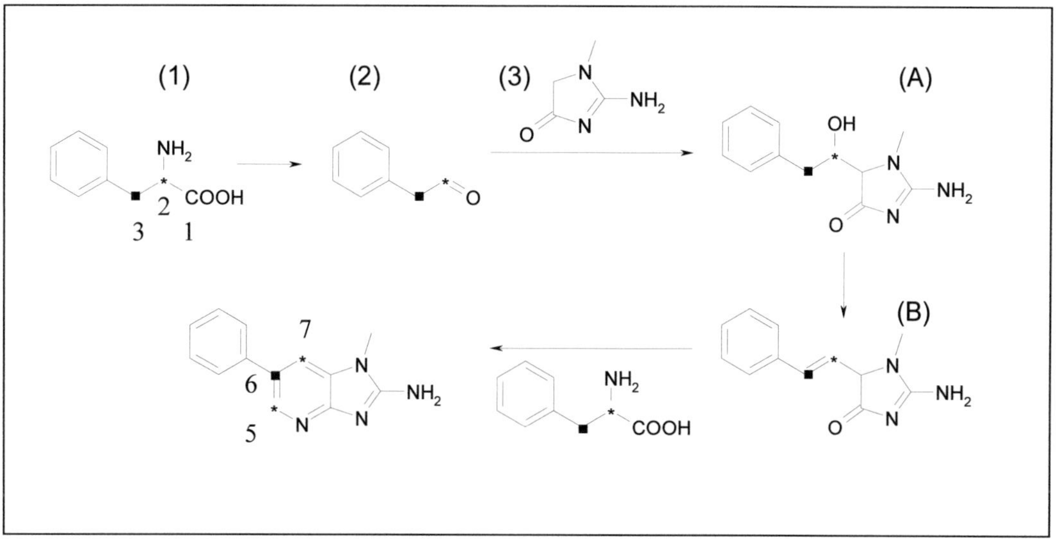

Fig. 4. Formation of PhIP. The marked carbon atoms correspond to the labelled positions in the experiments. Intermediate reaction products are signalled. Adapted from Murkovic et al. (Murkovic et al., 1999; Murkovic, 2004).

2.1 Parameters affecting the yield of HCAs

Among the different parameters affecting the formation of HCAs, temperature is the most important. The levels of HCAs are highly dependent on the temperature of the cooking process. In general, the amounts of HCAs increase at high temperature (Knize et al., 1994; Skog et al., 1995, 1997). Thus, HCAs form primarily in the crust of the cooked products and to a lesser extent in the inner part, which is where the temperature is lower (Skog et al., 1995).

Heat and mass transfer are variables that affect the formation of HCAs in cooking processes. Heating of meat produces protein denaturation, losses of fat and moisture and changes in the shrinkage and porosity of the meat or fish matrix. When heat is applied to the surface of the meat, it is transferred to the centre, creating a temperature gradient between the surface and the centre. As the temperature at the surface increases, the partial pressure of water increases at the surface, which causes a vapour flow towards the centre, where it condenses and releases heat. The increase of water content at the centre produces a flow of water towards the surface, even out of the meat (Persson et al., 2002). This water transport brings precursors of HCAs to the surface of the meat and to the drippings. In consequence, heat from the hot source favours the reaction between precursors of HCAs, and therefore HCAs can be found in drippings, even at higher amounts than in the food itself (Skog et al., 1997; Pais et al., 1999). Mechanisms controlling heat and mass transfer during thermal processing of beefburgers were studied by Bea. Kovácsné in a doctoral thesis at Lund University (B. Kovácsné, 2004). Cooking methods involve different heat and mass flows. Roasting entails transference of heat by convection through the air and radiation through the walls. In cooking methods where liquid surrounds the meat, such as stewing, boiling or deep-frying, heat is transferred by convection. Pan-frying produces heat transference to the meat by conduction and convection through a layer of fat and water. In contact frying, the temperature in the outermost part of the meat does not rise above 100ºC as long as water is present, and from the crust to a certain depth there is an evaporation zone. When crust is formed, heat flow towards the inside of the meat slows down because the crust insulates to some extent. Likewise, coating foods can reduce the formation of HCAs due to the insulating effect of the coating, and conductive heat transfer dominates inside the meat (Busquets et al., 2008; Persson et al., 2002; Skog et al., 2003). In general, roasting, boiling, stir-frying and stewing are the cooking methods in which lower amount of HCAs are formed; whereas griddling, pan-frying, barbecuing and deep-frying are the methods that lead to higher levels of HCAs, due to greater heat transfer (Busquets et al., 2004, 2008; Sinha et al., 1998a, 1998b; Skog et al., 1998). An example of the profile of temperatures when frying meat is shown in Fig. 5. Chicken breasts fillets, 1 cm in thickness, were fried in an aluminium frying pan, without adding fat, at 220 °C for 5 minutes each site. K-type thermocouples were inserted in different sites of the fillet; 2 in the centre of the fillet (T centre 1, 2); two were fixed at 1 mm below the upper and the lower surface (T surface 1,2), and one thermocouple was placed between the pan surface and the fillet to measure the temperature (Frying T), which was recorded every 10 seconds. The temperature profile measured was found highly reproducible when frying different fillets evidencing that the heat and mass transfer mechanisms taking place during the cooking process are reproducible. The temperature in the centre of the fillet did not go over 100 °C and the temperature at 1 mm below the surface never reached the frying temperature.

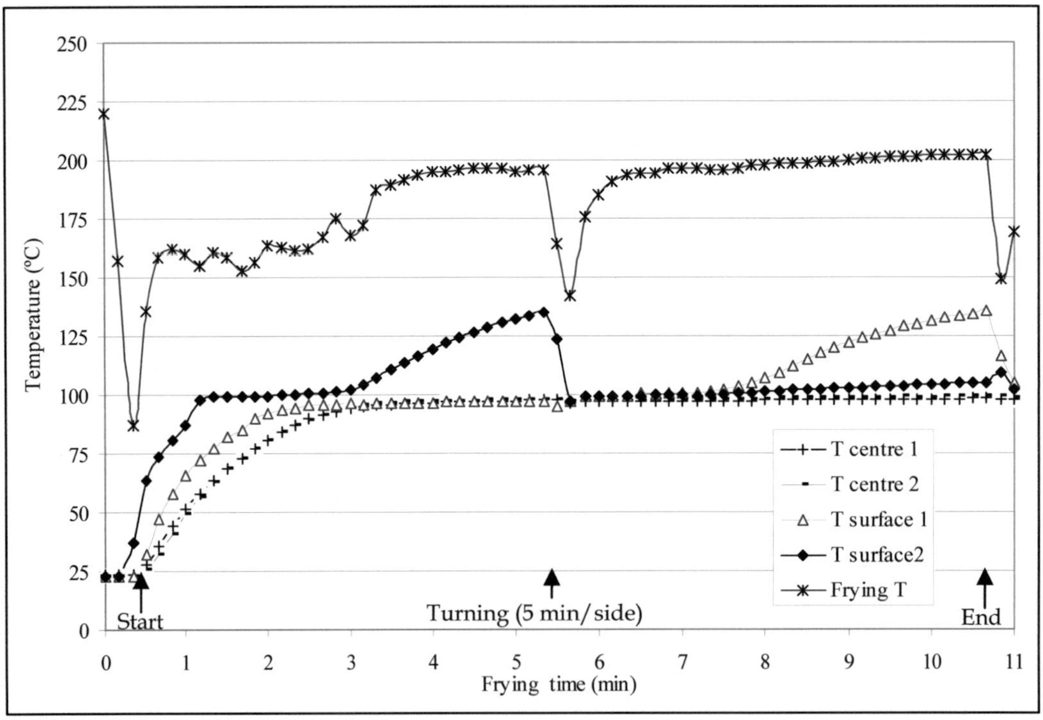

Fig. 5. Temperature profiles during pan-frying of a chicken fillet (1cm thick). Each side of the fillet was in contact with the hot surface for 5 minutes. The temperature of the pan was set at 220 °C.

Knowledge on the physical mechanisms affecting the formation of HCAs has led researchers to look for ways to decrease the formation of these mutagens. Changing cooking practices to minimize weight loss resulted in less formation of HCAs because of the alteration of the mass transfer of HCA precursors. The addition of NaCl, sodium tryphosphate or carbohydrates with water-holding capacity to meat prior to cooking was an efficient and simple way to reduce the subsequent formation of HCAs, explained by a reduction in the transport of water-soluble precursors towards the crust (Persson et al., 2003, 2004). Based on the same principle, microwaving beef patties before frying caused a reduction in mutagenicity possibly due to the loss of water and HCA precursors during the pre-treatment (Felton et al., 1994). Flipping the food frequently reduced the formation of HCAs because the meat has spent less time in contact with the hot surface (Salmon et al., 2000; Tran et al., 2002); and shortening cooking time or lowering cooking temperature also resulted in lower heat and mass transfer. As a result of the above-mentioned studies, easy-to-adopt cooking practices that reduce exposure to HCAs can be recommended.

Alternatively, solutions can also be found interfering in the chemical reactions leading to the formation of HCAs. For instance, one of the most effective methods reported for the inhibition of the formation of PhIP has been marinating the meat with red wine previous to the cooking process involving heat, effect that was markedly different to control marinades containing water and ethanol (Busquets et al., 2006). An example of the reduction of PhIP in fried chicken with marinating time is shown in Fig. 6.

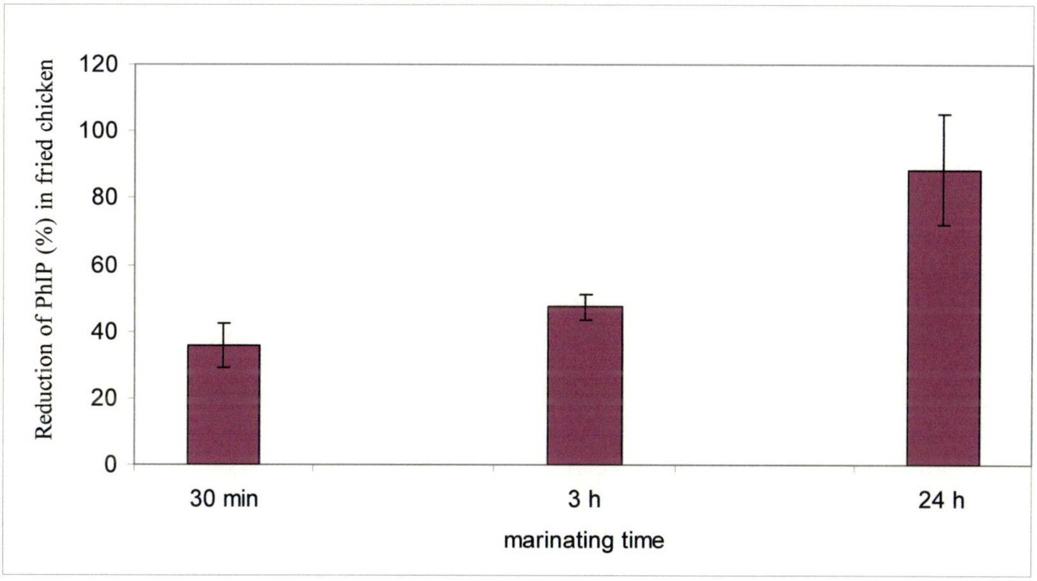

Fig. 6. Effect of marinating time on the reduction of PhIP in fried chicken. The marinating media was red wine. The wine characterisation and experimental conditions are as reported in Busquets et al. 2006.

One way to interfere in the formation of HCAs is using antioxidants, which may affect radical reactions involved in the formation of HCAs by scavenging free radicals (Kikugawa, 1999). Antioxidants have been shown to exert both anti- and pro-oxidative effects, depending on their concentration and type. For instance, Johansson and Jägerstad studied the effect of several antioxidants, at different concentrations, on the formation of HCAs in model systems. The results showed that, surprisingly, most antioxidants increased the formation of HCAs and that the rate of the effect depended on the concentration. Likewise, a lack of correlation was found between the concentration of the antioxidant and the effect observed (Johansson & Jägerstad, 1996). In summary, the formation of the heterocyclic amines which mechanism of formation may involve radical reactions can be enhanced or reduced depending on the particular cooking conditions used. Therefore, the effect of antioxidants on the formation of HCAs is not clear yet (Balogh et al., 2000; Britt et al., 1998; Melo 2008; Murkovic et al., 1998; Oguri et al., 1998; Shin et al., 2002; Tai et al., 2001; Tsen et al., 2006).

2.2 Levels of HCAs in food

Nowadays it is accepted that the main source of exposure to HCAs is the intake of cooked meat and fish. In order to know the type and amounts of HCAs to which humans are exposed, the content of HCAs has been determined in a high number of food items and the reported amounts are compiled periodically (Felton et al. 2000; Layton et al., 1995; Skog et al., 1998). To date about 20 mutagenic HCAs have been identified in cooked proteinaceous food and new ones may be identified in the future; species which structure is close to HCAs, if not HCAs, have been detected recently (Busquets et al., 2008). The most commonly found HCAs in thermally treated proteinaceous food are shown in Fig. 7.

To have an overview on the amount of HCAs in commonly consumed food items, the concentration of HCAs in over 20 publications have been summarized in Fig. 8 (Ahn et al 2005; Bermudo et al., 2005 ; Borgen et al., 2004; Busquets et al., 2004, 2006, 2008; Casal et al., 2004; Cheng et al., 2007; Gerbl et al., 2004; Khan et al., 2008; Lan et al., 2004; Melo et al., 2008; Ni et al., 2008; Oz et al., 2007; Persson et al., 2004; Ristic et al. 2004; Salmon et al., 2006; Toribio et al., 2007; Tsen et al., 2006; Warzecha et al., 2004; Wong et al, 2005). The average concentrations of several HCAs in meats cooked using different methods shows that chicken presents the highest concentration of HCAs, and in particular of the amines called DMIP and PhIP, which are structurally related, and the comutagens and neurotoxic amines harman and norharman, which were also found at relative high concentrations in venison. For a review on the latter ones, see Pfau & Skog (2004). The higher abundance of PhIP and DMIP in chicken can be due to the higher amount of some free amino acids such as phenylalanine mainly but also tyrosine, leucine, isoleucine or threonine, whereas the lower content identified in other meats can be due to the lower content of sugars or creatine/creatinine (Bjeldanes et al., 1982; Jägerstad et al., 1983a, 1983b ; Khan et al., 2009). Cooking methods also play an important role in the formation of PhIP because low amounts of this usually abundant amine have also been quantified in fried chicken breast cooked in the Chinese style (Wong et al., 2005; Salmon et al., 2006). Interestingly, low content of PhIP, below 2 ng/g, was found in turkey cooked by a prolonged frying process (15 min/side at 190-200°C) (Warzecha et al., 2004). Pork showed the highest content of the HCAs named IQ, MeIQx, 4,8-DiMeIQx, Trp-P-2 and Trp-P-1, and any HCA stand out in beef samples in terms of concentration level. The median concentration of HCAs in beef was below 3 ng/g; and even lower amounts were quantified in fish. Compared with previous data (Layton et al., 1995; Skog et al., 1998; Felton et al., 2000), the amounts of HCAs determined in fish for the studied period are low. The cause of this low occurrence may be the oriental recipies used, which use ingredients with antioxidant properties and cooking methods with low heat transfer (Wong et al., 2005; Salmon et al., 2006). The data in the papers included in Fig. 8 corroborates that the cooking methods involving higher heat transfer (barbecuing, frying, griddling and grilling) are related to higher levels of HCAs, whereas the processes with lower heat transfer (stewing, stir-frying, roasting, coated-frying and boiling) are related to lower amounts of HCAs.

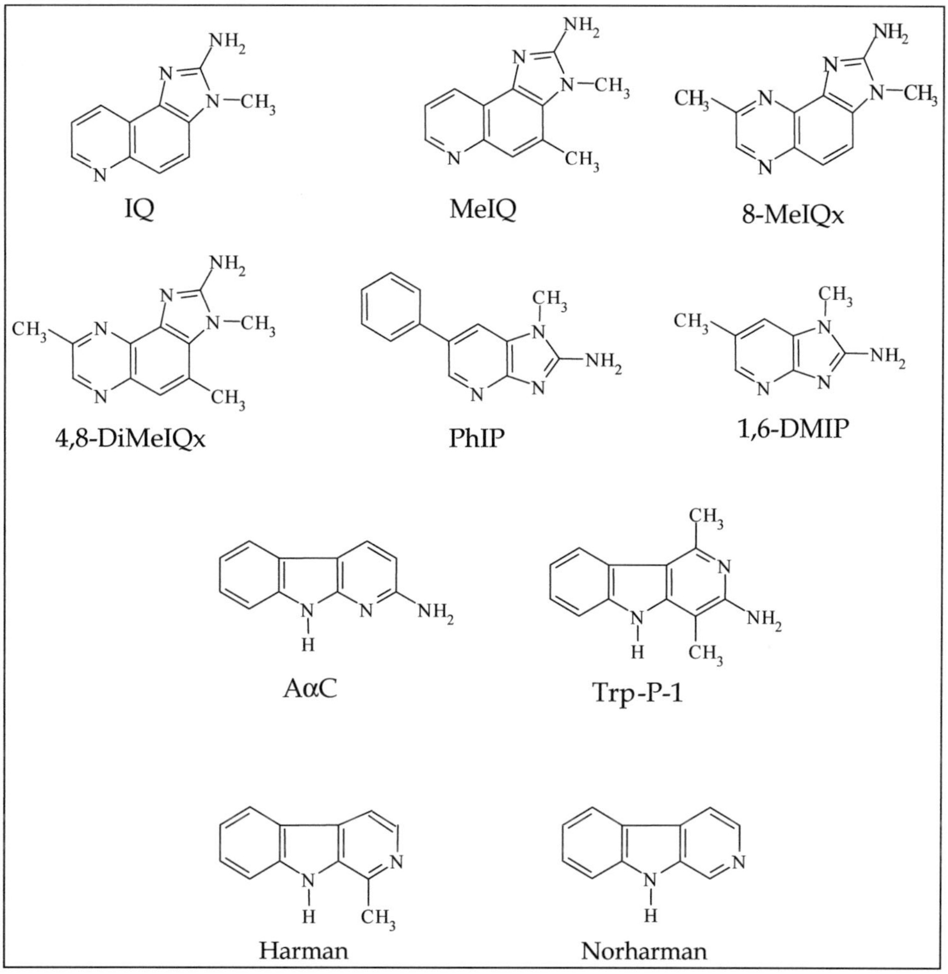

Fig. 7. Chemical structure of HCAs commonly found in cooked protein rich food.

2.3 Assessment of the exposure to HCAs

The toxicological effect of the habitual exposure of HCAs on humans is still unknown. There are two main approaches to quantifying exposure to HCAs; the first one evaluates the correlation between the intake of HCAs and increased risk of different types of human cancer; the second, searches for biomarkers of exposure to HCAs in biological fluids that correlate with the final molecule causing DNA damage. However analytical methodology for the analysis of such biomarkers under a normal exposure to HCAs is at its initial stages (Busquets et al., 2009; Frandsen et al., 2002, 2007, 2008); a few biomarker of exposure have been proposed so far but their analysis and correlation with cancer incidence in large cohorts has not been carried out yet, to the best of our knowledge.

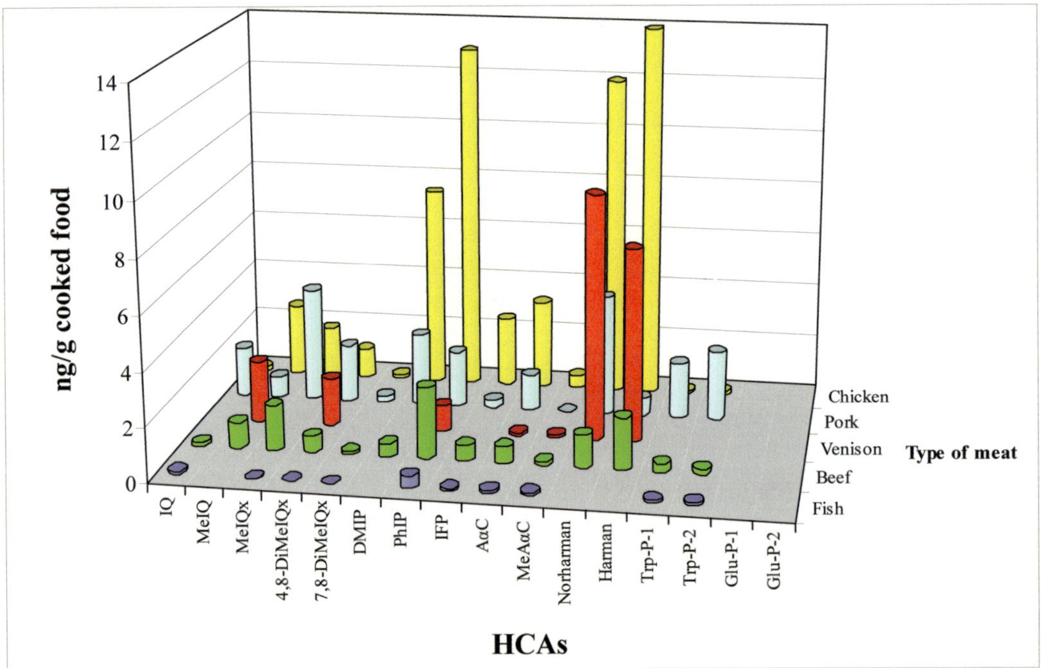

Fig. 8. Concentration of HCAs, identified by their acronym, reported in chicken, pork, venison, beef and fish items cooked in various ways.

Epidemiological studies relate the content of specific HCAs in food and the incidence of particular types of cancer. Several epidemiological studies have found a positive correlation between the intake of some HCAs and different types of human cancer (Butler et al., 2003; Cross A.J et at., 2011; Destefani et al., 1997, 1998; Martinez et al., 2007; Sinha et al., 2001) whereas other studies have found no such correlation (Augustsson et al., 1999; Gunter et al., 2005; Sonestedt et al., 2008). Numerous factors hinder reaching conclusions on the association of HCAs and human cancer by means of dietary calculations. Problems still to be surmounted are: the difficulty in getting accurate information on eating habits; bias, inconsistent reporting or misclassification; the fact that different cooking methods and degrees of doneness cause very different HCA content, as discussed earlier in this chapter; difficulty in quantifying cooking doneness using questionnaires; difficulty in considering variations in day-to-day diet; the existence of multiple HCAs and possibly some other factors that have not yet been identified. The representativity of the food analysed and the accuracy of HCA quantification must also be taken into account. For instance, several studies have related the occurrence of MeIQx or 4,8-DiMeIQx with cancer but these amines occur at low concentration, usually <2 ng/g cooked food, as it is shown in Figure 8, and their determination is difficult and possibly it is carried out with low accuracy. In addition, the whole amount of the HCAs ingested is not bioavailable, in part due to other components of the meal, but epidemiologic studies can not take these unknown parameters into consideration. Furthermore, only a fraction of the bioavailable HCAs are activated to the ultimate electrophilic intermediate that causes the genetic damage and this activation can be more or less effective depending on the phenotypes of the enzymes involved in the activation pathways and on lifestyle factors (Le Marchand et al., 2001). Moreover, there are mechanisms in the human body that repair mutations and, in addition, the mutations that initiate cancer processes may be caused by environmental factors other than HCAs in diet. Another factor, not unique to HCAs, is that the delay between the evaluation of the exposure and disease outcome (Alexander et al., 2002). These factors show that there is a big gap between the estimation of HCA exposure and the identification of the origin of cancer processes by means of epidemiologic studies.

Regardless of all the existing limitations and approximations necessary to asses the exposure to HCAs, the individual daily exposure to HCAs has been quantified in several countries. For Asian populations: 50 ng in China (Wong et al., 2005) and 72 ng in Japan (Kobayashi et al., 2002) were estimated. In general, higher values have been found for European populations: 69 ng in Germany (Rohrmann et al., 2007); 160 ng (Augustsson et al., 1997), 690 ng (Ericson et al. 2007) and 520 ng (Sonestedt et al., 2008) in Sweden; 330 ng in Switzerland (Zimmerli et al., 2001); and 286 ng (Busquets et al., 2008) and 606 ng in Spain (Busquets et al., 2004). Several studied performed in the United States studies found high values: 1.690 ng (Layton et al., 1995), 455 ng (Keating & Bogen, 2001), 585 ng (Bogen & Keating, 2001) and 715-1.293 ng (Keating & Bogen, 2004). The quoted intakes were calculated for an average body mass of 65 Kg. The levels of exposure estimated from food frequency questionnaires and analysis of HCAs in food may be useful in toxicological studies to define the impact of HCAs on health and to make risk-based recommendations about reducing exposure to HCAs. However, the reported values have to be used in full awareness of the intrinsic limitations of exposure assessment by means of food frequency questionnaires and determination of HCAs in a limited number of cooked foods.

The intake of HCAs is not directly related with mutations in the DNA. Only a part of the total amount of HCAs present in heated proteinaceous food will be absorbed. To the best of our knowledge, few studies have focused on the bioavailable or effective dose of HCAs, although this is key to assessing the effective dose of the dietary intake of HCAs. To understand the influence of digestion parameters on the release of HCAs, Kulp and coworkers used a model system to test the effect of several enzymes (amylase, pepsin and pancreatin) on the digestion of well-done chicken (Kulp et al., 2003) and pancreatin was the only enzyme that favoured the bioavailability of HCAs. In addition, HCAs differed greatly from each other in ways that affected their bioavailability; PhIP, which is less polar than the other amines studied, was 50% present in each fraction, which implies that PhIP is less accessible than more polar HCAs. Very important also was the finding that the higher the degree of doneness, the lower the bioavailability of HCAs was (Kulp et al., 2003). Another factor that may affect the bioavailability of HCAs is the presence of fibre in the meal. Experiments carried out in rats revealed that dietary fibre, 95% of which is contributed by whole plant cell walls, may protect by adsorbing carcinogens, thus lowering their effective concentration in the alimentary tract, and by carrying the carcinogens out of the body in faeces (Ferguson & Harris, 1996). However, not all types of fibre had adsorptive abilities. The most hydrophobic plant cell wall preparations containing the polymer suberin, which occur in the diet, for example in potato skins, showed the highest adsorption capacity for

HCAs among the fibre examined and preparations with lignin showed intermediate adsorptive abilities. The adsorption of HCAs to the plant cell walls increased with increasing hydrophobicity of the HCA (Ferguson et al., 1995; Ferguson & Harris, 1996; Harris et al., 1996; Hayatsu et al., 1993b). Similarly, chlorophyllin, intestinal microflora and certain bacterial strains contained in fermented foods may decrease the bioavailability of HCAs by direct binding of HCAs to their structure (Hayatsu et al., 1993a; Kassie et al., 2001, 2004; Knasmüller et al., 2001; Orrhage et al., 1994; 2002).

Once the HCAs are bioavailable, they require metabolic activation to damage DNA. Most HCAs are oxidized in the body and just a small portion is excreted unchanged. The first step to activate HCAs is catalyzed by cytochrome P450 enzymes (CYP). 57 CYP genes have been identified in human genome, half of which are involved in xenobiotic metabolism (Glatt, 2006). Among the different CYPs, those of family 1 have been found to participate in the metabolism of HCAs. CYP1A2 shows the highest activity for N-hydroxylation or activation of the HCAs to the ultimate mutagenic specie (Boobis et al., 1994; Glatt, 2006; Rich et al., 1992; Zhao et al., 1994). CYP1A2 activity may vary from person to person and can be activated by lifestyle factors such as smoking or eating habits (Lang et al., 1994). N-hydroxylated HCAs undergo O-acetylation and O-sulphatation catalyzed by N-acetyltransferases and sulphotransferases, respectively. These esters are hydrolyzed to produce highly electrophilic arylnitrenium ions, considered to be the final genotoxicants, which react with some sites of the DNA. The reactive nitrenium ion also reacts with proteins (Buonarati et al., 1990; Turesky et al., 1992; Turesky et al., 2004). Detoxification involves converting the toxicants to polar molecules that can be excreted or transported to extrahepatic tissues. Various detoxification pathways, such as ring hydroxylation, catalyzed by CYPs, or glucoronidation, catalyzed by UDP-glucoronosyltransferases, compete with the activation routes. Understanding the metabolic pathways of HCAs and developing analytical methodology capable of determining metabolites from HCAs in biological fluids with high accuracy, despite their low concentration and complexity of the matrices, is providing the tools to identify species that could be proved to be biomarkers of exposure. The analysis of species proved to be biomakers of exposure to HCAs in large cohorts and its relation with cancer incidence will be ultimate evidence to relate HCAs with human cancer.

3. Conclusion

Heat treatments applied during cooking processes cause the formation of mutagenic compounds from the reaction of natural precursors present in raw food. Although the exposure to such toxicants seems unavoidable, it can be highly reduced by just applying minor changes in cooking and eating habits. The exposure to HCAs is currently being estimated with methods comprising many approximations. Different types and levels of food borne mutagens are present in frequently eaten food items. The bioavailability of these cooking mutagens, their metabolic activation and DNA repair mechanism are also variable. The pathogenesis can also be caused by other factors, and it appears with a delay on time with respect to the causes that induced the genetic damage. For these reasons, the link between food borne mutagens and cancer has not been well established in humans although the effect of high concentrations of the mutagens in animals has shown to cause tumours. The mortality rate of cancer, the economical burden that the disease represents, and the evidences on the exposure to food borne mutagens discussed in this chapter, claim major attention from the legislative bodies, which should establish maximum concentration limits for these species in commercial food products and recommend guidelines for "good cooking practices". Legislation on this topic would encourage the food industry to monitor, control and ultimately reduce the exposure food borne mutagens. Besides, the public health institutions and scientist should inform the population about the existence of the food borne mutagens and ways to minimise their formation. A change towards healthier eating/cooking habits in terms of exposure to cooking toxicants may be fomented with the approach used when disseminating the information. If the exposure is presented as something unavoidable, the consummers will resing themselves and do nothing. However, the attitude from the public may be more active if they receive information in a positive way; there is exposure to hazardous compounds but it can be reduced easily by using certain practices such as cooking methods with low heat transfer (boiling, stewing, coating, flipping the food frequently); lowering cooking time and temperature or using ingredients that interfer in the Maillard reaction. Once individuals are aware of the problem and willing to solve it, these generates a commercial opportunity, and for the first time companies would invest in products for a diet with low in food borne toxicants without being pushed to it. In summary, food borne carcinogens are not a dead end; individuals, food companies and public bodies have health or business interest in them.

4. Acknowledgement

The author acknowledges the researchers in the CECEM group (University of Barcelona); Mutagenlab (Lund University); the Nanosicence and Nanotechnology group and the Biomaterials group (University of Brighton). Dr. Lubinda Mbundi (University of Brighton) is acknowledged for interesting discussions.

5. References

Ahn, J. & Gruen, I.U. (2005). Heterocyclic amines: 2. Inhibitory effects of natural extracts on the formation of polar and nonpolar heterocyclic amines in cooked beef. *J.Food Sci.,70*, C263-C268.

Alexander, J.; Reistad, R.; Hegstad, S.; Frandsen, H.; Ingebrigtsen, K.; Paulsen, J.E. & Becher, G. (2002).Biomarkers of exposure to heterocyclic amines:approaches to improve the exposure assessment. Food Chem.Toxicol., 40, pp. 1131-1137.

Altaki, M.S; Santos, F.J. & Galceran, M.T. (2011). Occurrence of furan in coffee from Spanish market: contribution of brewing and roasting. *Food Chem.*, Vol. *126*, pp. 1527-1532.

Ames, B.N.; McCann, J. & Yamasaki; E. (1975). Methods for detecting carcinogens and mutagens with the salmonella/mammalian-microsome mutagenicity test. *Mutat.Res., 31*, pp. 347-363.

Arnoldi, A.; Corain, E.A.; Scaglioni, L. & Ames, J.M. (1997). New Colored Compounds from the Maillard Reaction between xylose and lysine. *J. Agric. Food Chem.*, Vol. *45*, pp. 650-655.

Augustsson, K.; Skog, K; Jägerstad, M. & Steineck, G. (1997). Assessment of the Human Exposure to Heterocyclic Amines. *Carcinogenesis*, Vol. 18, pp. 1931-1935.

Augustsson, K.; Skog, K.; Jägerstad, M.; Dickman, P.W. & Steineck, G. (1999). Dietary Heterocyclic Amines and Cancer of the Colon, Rectum, Bladder, and Kidney - A Population-Based Study. *Lancet*, Vol. 353, pp. 703-707.

Balogh, Z.; Gray, J.I.; Gomaa, E.A. & Booren, A.M. (2000). Formation and Inhibition of Has in fried Ground Beef Patties. *Food Chem.Toxicol.*, Vol. 38, pp. 395-401.

Bermudo, E.; Ruiz-Calero, V.; Puignou, L. & Galceran, M.T. (2005). Analysis of heterocyclic amines in chicken by liquid chromatography with electrochemical detection. *Anal. Chim. Acta*, Vol. *536*, pp. 83-90.

Bermudo, E.; Moyano, E.; Puignou, L. & Galceran, M.T. (2006). Determination of acrylamide in foodstuffs by liquid chromatography ion-trap tandem mass-spectrometry using an improved clean-up procedure. *Anal.Chim.Acta* Vol. 559, pp. 207-214.

Bjeldanes, L.F.; Morris, M.M.; Felton, J.S.; Healy, S.; Stuermer, D.; Berry, P.; Timourian, H. & Hatch, F.T. (1982). Mutagens from the cooking of food. III. Survey by Ames/Salmonella test of mutagen formation in secondary sources of cooked dietary protein. *Food Chem Toxicol.*, 20, pp. 365-369.

Boobis, A.R.; Lynch, A.M.; Murray, S.; Delatorre, R.; Solans, A.; Farre, M.; Segura, J.; Gooderham, N.J. & Davies, D.S. (1994). CYP1A2-catalyzed conversion of dietary heterocyclic amines to their proximate carcinogens is their major route of metabolism in humans. *Cancer Res.*, Vol. 54, pp. 89-94.

Borgen, E. & Skog, K. (2004). Heterocyclic amines in some Swedish cooked foods industrially prepared or from fast food outlets and restaurants. *Mol.Nutr.Food Res.*, Vol. 48, pp. 292-298.

Britt, C.; Gomaa, E.A.; Gray, J.I. & Booren, A.M. (1998). Influence of cherry tissue on lipid oxidation and heterocyclic aromatic amine formation in ground beef patties. *J. Agric. Food Chem.*, Vol. 46, pp. 4891-4897.

Buonarati, M.H.; Turteltaub, K.W.; Shen, N.H. & Felton, J.S. (1990). Role of sulfation and acetylation in the activation of 2-hydroxyamino-1-methyl-6-phenylimidazo[4,5-b]pyridine to intermediates which bind DNA. *Mutat.Res.*, Vol. 245, pp. 185-190.

Busquets, R.; Bordas, M.; Toribio, F.; Puignou, L. & Galceran, M.T. (2004). Occurrence of heterocyclic amines in several home-cooked meat dishes of the Spanish diet. *J. Chromatogr. B*, Vol. 802, pp. 79-86.

Busquets, R.; Puignou, L.; Galceran, M.T. & Skog, K. (2006). Effect of red wine marinades on the formation of heterocyclic amines in fried chicken breast. *J. Agric. Food Chem.*, 54, pp. 8376-8384.

Busquets, R.; Puignou, L.; Galceran, M.T.; Wakabayashi, K. & Skog, K. (2007). Liquid Chromatography tandem mass spectrometry analysis of 2-amino-1-methyl-6-(4-hydroxyphenyl)imidazo[4,5- *b*]pyridine in cooked meats. *J. Agric. Food Chem.*, Vol. 55, pp. 9318-9324.

Busquets, R.; Mitjans, D.; Puignou, L. & Galceran, M.T. (2008). Quantification of heterocyclic amines from thermally processed meats selected from a small-scale population-based study. *Mol.Nutr. Food Res.*, Vol. *52*, pp. 1408-1420.

Busquets, R.; Jönsson, J. Å.; Frandsen, H.; Puignou, L.; Galceran, M.T. & Skog, K. (2009). Hollow-fibre supported liquid membrane extraction and LC-MS/MS detection for the analysis of heterocyclic amines in urine samples. *Mol. Nutr. Food Res.*, Vol. 53, pp. 1496-1504.

Butler, L.M.; Sinha, R.; Millikan, R.C.; Martin, C.F.; Newman, B.; Gammon, M.D.; Ammerman, A.S. & Sandler, R.S.(2003). Heterocyclic amines, meat intake, and association with colon cancer in a population-based study. *Amer.J.Epidemiol.*, Vol. 157, pp. 434-445.

Casal, S.; Mendes, E.; Fernandes, J.O.; Oliveira, M.B.P.P.; & Ferreira, M.A. (2004). Analysis of heterocyclic aromatic amines in foods by gas chromatography-mass spectrometry as their tert.- butyldimethylsilyl derivatives. *J. Chromatogr. A*, Vol. 1040, 105-114.

Cheng, K.W.; Wu, Q.; Zheng, Z.P.; Peng, X.; Simon, J.E.; Chen, F.; & Wang, M. (2007). Inhibitory Effect of Fruit Extracts on the Formation of Heterocyclic Amines. *J. Agric. Food Chem.*, Vol. 55, pp. 10359-10365.

Commoner, B.; Vithayathil, A.J.; Dolara, P.; Nair, S.; Madyastha, P. & Cuca, G.C. (1978). Formation of mutagens in beef and beef extract during cooking. *Science*, Vol. 201, pp. 913-916.

Chung, S.Y.; Yettella, R.R.; Kim, J.S.; Kwon, K.; Kim, M.C.;. & Min D.B. (2011). Effects of grilling and roasting on the levels of polycyclic aromatic hydrocarbons in beef and pork. *Food Chem.*, Vol. 129, pp. 1420-1426.

Cross, A.J., Freedman, Nl D., Ren,J., Ward, M. H., Hollenbeck, A. R., Schatzkin,A, Sinha, R., & Abnet, C.C. (2011). Meat consumption and risk of esophageal and gastric cancer in a large prospective study. *Am.J.Gastroenterol.*, Vol. 106, pp. 432-442.

Destefani, E.; Ronco, A.; Mendilaharsu, M.; Guidobono, M. & Deneopellegrini, H. (1997). Meat Intake, Heterocyclic Amines, and Risk of Breast-Cancer - A Case-Control Study in Uruguay. *Cancer Epidem.Biomarker.Prev.*, Vol. 6, pp. 573-581.

Destefani, E.; Ronco, A.; Mendilaharsu, M. & Deneopellegrini, H. (1998). Case-Control Study on the Role of Heterocyclic Amines in the Etiology of Upper Aerodigestive Cancers in Uruguay. *Nutr.Cancer*, Vol. 32, pp. 43-48.

Drabik-Markiewicz,. G.; Dejaegher, B.; De Mey, E.; Kowalska, T.; Paelinck, H.; & Heyden Vander Y. (2011). Influence of putrescine, cadaverine, spermidine or spermine on the formation of N-nitrosamine in heated cured pork meat. *Food Chem.*, Vol. 126, pp. 1539-1545.

Druckrey, H. & Preussmann, R. (1962). The formation of carcinogenic nitrosamines, for example, in tobacco smoke. *Naturwissenschaften.*, Vol. 49, pp. 498-499.

Ericson, U.; Wirfält, E.; Mattisson, I.; Gullberg, B. & Skog, K. (2007). Dietary intake of heterocyclic amines in relation to socio-economic, lifestyle and other dietary factors: estimates in a Swedish population. *Public Health Nutr.*, Vol. 10, pp. 616-627.

Felton, J.S.; Fultz, E.; Dolbeare, F.A. and Knize, M.G. (1994). Effect of microwave pretreatment on heterocyclic aromatic amine mutagens/carcinogens in fried beef patties. *Food Chem.Toxicol.* , Vol. *32*, pp. 897-903.

Felton, J.S.; Jägerstad, M.; Knize, M.G.; Skog, K.; & Wakabayashi, K. (2000). Content in Foods, Beverages and Tobacco. In: *Food Borne Carcinogens*, Nagao M, Sugimura T (Eds), pp. 31-71, JohnWiley & Sons Ltd.-VCH, ISBN 9780471983996, Weinheim.

Ferguson, L.R.; Roberton, A.M.; Watson, M.E.; Triggs, C.M. & Harris, P.J. (1995).The Effects of a Soluble-Fiber Polysaccharide on the Adsorption of Carcinogens to Insoluble Dietary-Fibers. *Chem.Biol.Inter.*, Vol. 95, pp. 245-255.

Ferguson, L.R. & Harris, P.J. Studies on the Role of Specific Dietary-Fibers in Protection Against Colorectal-Cancer. *Mutat.Res.Fundam.Mol.Mech.Mut.* 1996, *350*, 173-184.

Frandsen, H.; Frederiksen, H. & Alexander, J. (2002). 2-amino-1-methyl-6-(5-hydroxy-)phenylimidazo[4,5-*b*]pyridine (5-OH-PhIP), a biomarker for the genotoxic dose of the heterocyclic amine, 2-amino-1-methyl-6-phenylimidazo[4,5-*b*]pyridine (PhIP). *Food Chem. Toxicol.*, Vol. 40, pp. 1125-1130.

Frandsen, H. Deconjugation of N-glucoronide conjugated metabolites with hydrazine hydrate-Biomarkers for exposure to the food-borne carcinogen 2-amino-1-methyl-6-phenylimidazo[4,5-b]pyridine(PhIP). (2007).*Food Chem. Toxicol.*, Vol. 45, pp. 863-870.

Frandsen, H. (2008). Biomonitoring of urinary metabolites of 2-amino-1-methyl-6-phenylimidazo[4,5-b]pyridine (PhIP) following human consumption of cooked chicken. *Food Chem. Toxicol.*, Vol. 46, pp. 3200-3205.

Frandsen, H.; Frederiksen, H. & Alexander J. (2002). 2-amino-1-methyl-6-(5-hydroxy-) phenylimidazo[4,5- *b*]pyridine (5-OH-PhIP), a biomarker for the genotoxic dose of the heterocyclic amine, 2-amino-1-methyl-6-phenylimidazo[4,5-*b*]pyridine (PhIP). *Food Chem. Toxicol.*, 40, pp. 1125-1130.

Gerbl, U.; Cichna, M.; Zsivkovits, M.; Knasmüller, S. & Sontag, G. (2004). Determination of heterocyclic aromatic amines in beef extract, cooked meat and rat urine by liquid chromatography with coulometric electrode array detection. *J.Chromatogr.B, 802*, pp. 107-113.

Glatt, H. & Sommer, Y. (2006). Health risks of 5-hydroxy-methyl-furfural (HMF) and related comounds, In: *Acrylamide and Other Hazardous Compounds in Heat-Treated Foods*, Skog, K., Alexander J. (Eds.), pp. 328-357, Woodhead Publishing Limited and CRC Press LLC, ISBN 1-84569-01107, Cambridge and Boca Raton.

Gunter, M.J.; Probst-Hensch, N.M.; Cortessis, V.K.; Kulldorff, M.; Haile, R.W. & Sinha, R. (2005).Meat intake, cooking-related mutagens and risk of colorectal adenoma in a sigmoidoscopy-based case-control study. *Carcinogenesis*, Vol. 26, pp. 637-642.

Harris, P.J.; Triggs, C.M.; Roberton, A.M.; Watson, M.E. & Ferguson, L.R. (1996). The Adsorption of Heterocyclic Aromatic-Amines by Model Dietary- Fibers with Contrasting Compositions. *Chem.Biol.Inter.*, Vol. 100, pp. 13-25.

Hayatsu, H. & Hayatsu, T. (1993a)Suppressing Effect of Lactobacillus-Casei Administration on the Urinary Mutagenicity Arising from Ingestion of Fried Ground- Beef in the Human. *Cancer Lett.*, Vol. 73, pp. 173-179.

Hayatsu, H.; Negishi, T.; Arimoto, S. & Hayatsu, T. (1993b). Porphyrins as Potential Inhibitors Against *Exposure to Carcinogens and Mutagens. Mutat.Res.*, Vol. 290, pp. *79-85.*

IARC Monographs on the evaluation of carcinogenic risks to humans. Some natural occurring substances: food items and constituents. Heterocyclic amines and mycotoxins. (1993). International Agency for Research on Cancer, Vol. 56, pp. 163-242, Lyon.

IARC Acrylamide. IARC Monographs on the Evaluation of Carcinogenic Risks to Humans. (1994). International Agency for Research on Cancer, pp. 389, Lyon.

IARC IARC Monographs on the evaluation of carcinogenic risks to humans. Dry cleaning, some chlorinated solvents, and other industrial chemicals. (1995). International Agency for Research on Cancer, Lyon 63, 393.

IARC- World Health Organzation. IARC classifies radiofrequency electromagnetic fields as possibly carcinogenic to humans. Press release 208. 31 May 2011.

Jägerstad, M.; Reuterswärd, A.L.; Öeste, R.; Dahlqvist, A.; Grivas, S.; Olsson, K. & Nyhammar, T. (1983a). Creatinine and Maillard reaction products as precursors of mutagenic compounds formed in fried beef. ACS Symp. Ser., *215*, pp. 507-519.

Jägerstad, M., Laser Reuterswaerd, A., Olsson, R., Grivas, S., Nyhammar, T., Olsson, K., & Dahlqvist, A. (1983b). Creatin(in)e and Maillard reaction products as precursors of mutagenic compounds: effects of various amino acids. *Food Chem.*, Vol. 12, pp. 255-264.

Johansson, M.A.E. & Jägerstad, M. (1996). Influence of pro-oxidants and antioxidants on the formation of mutagenic-carcinogenic heterocyclic amines in a model system. *Food Chem.*, Vol. 56, pp. 69-75.

Kassie, F.; Lhoste, E.F.; Bruneau, A.; Zsivkovits, M.; Ferk, F.; Uhl, M.; Zidek, T.; & Knasmüller, S. (2004). Effect of intestinal microfloras from vegetarians and meat eaters on the genotoxicity of 2-amino-3-methylimidazo[4,5-f]quinoline, a carcinogenic heterocyclic amine. *J.Chromatogr.B*, Vol. 802, pp. 211-215.

Kassie, F.; Rabot, S.; Kundi, M.; Chabicovsky, M.; Qin, H.M.; & Knasmüller, S. (2001). Intestinal microflora plays a crucial role in the genotoxicity of the cooked food mutagen 2-amino-3-*methylimidazo[4,5- f]quinoline (IQ).* Carcinogenesis, Vol. 22, pp. 1721-1725.

Keating, G.A. & Bogen, K.T. (2001). Methods for estimating heterocyclic amine concentrations in cooked meats in the US diet. *Food Chem.Toxicol.*, Vol. 39, pp. 29-43.

Keating, G.A. & Bogen, K.T. (2004). Estimates of heterocyclic amine intake in the US population. *J.Chromatogr.B,* Vol. 802, pp. 127-133.

Kulp, K.S.; Fortson, S.L.; Knize, M.G. & Felton, J.S.(2003).An in vitro model system to predict the bioaccessibility of heterocyclic amines from a cooked meat matrix. *Food Chem.Toxicol.*, Vol. 41, pp. 1701-1710.

Khan, M.R.; Busquets, R.; Santos, F.J. & Puignou, L.(2008).New method for the analysis of heterocyclic amines in meat extracts using pressurised liquid extraction and liquid chromatography-tandem mass spectrometry. J. Chromatogr. A, Vol. 1194, pp. 155-160.

Khan, M.R.; Bertus, L.M.; Busquets, R.; & Puignou, L. (2009). Mutagenic heterocyclic amine content in thermally processed offal products. *Food Chem.*, Vol. 112, pp. 838-843.

Kikugawa, K. (1999). Involvement of Free-Radicals in the Formation of Heterocyclic Amines and Prevention by Antioxidants. *Cancer Lett.*, Vol. 143, pp. 123-126.

Kovácsné, B. (2004). The mechanisms controlling heat and mass transfer on frying of beefburgers, Lund University. *Doctoral thesis.*

Knasmüller, S.; Steinkellner, H.; Hirschl, A.M.; Rabot, S.; Nobis, E.C. & Kassie, F. (2001). Impact of Bacteria in Dairy-Products and of the Intestinal Microflora on the Genotoxic and Carcinogenic Effects of Heterocyclic Aromatic-Amines. *Mutat.Res.Fundam.Mol.Mech.Mut.*, Vol. 480, pp. 129-138.

Knize, M.G.; Dolbeare, F.A.; Carroll, K.L.; Moore, D.H. & Felton, J.S. (1994). Effect of Cooking Time and Temperature on the Heterocyclic Amine Content of Fried Beef Patties. *Food Chem.Toxicol.,* Vol. 32, pp. 595-603.

Kobayashi, M.; Hanaoka, T.; Nishioka, S.; Kataoka, H. & Tsugane, S. (2002). Estimation of dietary HCA intakes in a large-scale population-based prospective study in Japan. *Mutat.Res.*, Vol. 506-507, pp. 233-241.

Lan, C.M.; Kao, T.H. & Chen, B.H. (2004).Effects of heating time and antioxidants on the formation of heterocyclic amines in marinated foods. *J.Chromatogr.B*, Vol. 802, pp. 27-37.

Lang, N.P.; Butler, M.A.; Massengill, J.; Lawson, M.; Stotts, R.C.; Hauerjensen, M. & Kadlubar, F.F. (1994). Rapid Metabolic Phenotypes for Acetyltransferase and Cytochrome P4501A2 and Putative Exposure to Food-Borne Heterocyclic Amines Increase the Risk for Colorectal-Cancer or Polyps. *Cancer Epidem.Biomarker.Prev.*, Vol. *3*, pp. 675-682.

Layton, D.W.; Bogen, K.T.; Knize, M.G.; Hatch, F.T.; Johnson, V.M. & Felton, J.S. (1995). Cancer Risk of Heterocyclic Amines in Cooked Foods - An Analysis and Implications for Research. *Carcinogenesis*, Vol. *16*, pp. 39-52.

Lezamiz, J.; Barri, T.; Jönsson, J.Å. & Skog, K. (2008). A simplified hollow-fibre supported liquid membrane extraction method for quantification of 2-amino-1-methyl-6-phenylimidazo[4,5-*b*]pyridine (PhIP) in urine and plasma samples. *Anal. Bioanal. Chem.*, Vol. *390*, pp. 689-696.

Lijinsky, W. & Shubik, B. (1964). Benzo[a]pyrene and other polynuclear hydrocarbons in charcoal-broiled meat. *Science (Washington, DC, United States)*. Vol. *145*, pp. 53-55.

Maga, J.A. (1979). Furans in foods. *Critical Reviews in Food Science and Nutrition*, Vol. *11*, pp. 355-400.

Martinez, M.E.; Jacobs, E.T.; Ashbeck, E.L.; Sinha, R.; Lance, P.; Alberts, D.S. and Thompson, P.A. (2007). Meat intake, preparation methods, mutagens and colorectal adenoma recurrence. *Carcinogenesis*, *28*, pp. 2019-2027.

Melo, A.; Viegas, O.; Eca, R.; Petisca, C.; Pinho, O.; & Ferreira, I.M.P.L. Extraction, Detection, and Quantification of Heterocyclic Aromatic Amines in Portuguese Meat Dishes by HPLC/Diode Array. (2008). *J.Liq.Chromatogr.Relat.Techno.*, Vol. *31*, pp. 772-787.

Mottram, D.S.; Wedzicha, B.L. & Dodson A.T. (2002). Acrylamide is formed in the Maillard reaction. *Nature*, Vol. *419*, 448-449.

Murkovic, M., Steinberger, D., & Pfannhauser, W. (1998). Antioxidant Spices Reduce the Formation of Heterocyclic Amines in Fried Meat. *Z.Lebensm.Unters.Forsch.A Foo.*, Vol. *207*, pp. 477-480.

Murkovic, M.; Weber, H.J.; Geiszler, S.; Frohlich, K. & Pfannhauser, W. (1999). Formation of the food associated carcinogen 2-amino-1-methyl-6-phenylimidazo[4,5-*b*]Pyridine (PhIP) in model systems. *Food Chem.*, Vol. *65*, pp. 233-237.

Murkovic, M. (2004). Formation of heterocyclic aromatic amines in model systems. *J. Chromatogr. B*, *802*, pp. 3-10.

Nagao, M.; Honda, M.; Seino, Y.; Yahagi, T. & Sugimura, T. (1977). Mutagenicities of smoke condensates and the charred surface of fish and meat. *Cancer Lett.*, Vol. *2*, pp. 221-226.

Ni, W.; McNaughton, L.; LeMaster, D.M.; Sinha, R.; & Turesky, R.J. (2008). Quantitation of 13 Heterocyclic Aromatic Amines in Cooked Beef, Pork, and Chicken by Liquid Chromatography-Electrospray Ionization/Tandem Mass Spectrometry. *J.Agric.Food Chem.*, Vol. *56*, pp. 68-78.

Oguri, A.; Suda, M.; Totsuka, Y.; Sugimura, T. & Wakabayashi, K. (1998). Inhibitory Effects of Antioxidants on Formation of Heterocyclic Amines. *Mutat. Res. Fundam. Mol. Mech. Mut.*, Vol. 402, pp. 237-245.

Orrhage, K.; Sillerstrom, E.; Gustafsson, J.A.; Nord, C.E. & Rafter, J. (1994). Binding of Mutagenic Heterocyclic Amines by Intestinal and Lactic-Acid Bacteria. *Mutat.Res.Fundam.Mol.Mech.Mut.*, Vol. 311, pp. 239-248.

Orrhage, K.M.; Annas, A.; Nord, C.E.; Brittebo, E.B. & Rafter, J.J. (2002). Effects of Lactic-Acid Bacteria on the Uptake and Distribution of the Food Mutagen Trp-P-2 in Mice. *Scand.J.Gastroenterol*, Vol. 37, pp. 215-221.

Oz, F.; Kaban, G. & Kaya, M. (2007). Effects of cooking methods on the formation of heterocyclic aromatic amines of two different species trout. *Food Chem., 104,* pp. 67-72.

Pais, P.; Salmon, C.P.; Knize, M.G. & Felton, J.S. (1999) Formation of mutagenic/carcinogenic heterocyclic amines in dry- heated model systems, meats, and meat drippings. *J. Agric. Food Chem.* Vol. *47,* pp. 1098-1108.

Persson, E.; Sjöholm, I. & Skog, K. (2002). Heat and mass transfer in chicken breasts: Effect on PhIP formation. *Eur.Food Res.Technol.*, Vol. 214, pp. 455-459.

Persson, E.; Sjöholm, I. & Skog, K. (2003). Effect of High Water-Holding Capacity on the Formation of Heterocyclic Amines in Fried Beefburgers. *J.Agric.Food Chem., Vol. 51,* pp. 4472-4477.

Persson, E.; Sjöholm, I.; Nyman, M. & Skog, K. (2004). Addition of Various Carbohydrates to Beef Burgers Affects the Formation of Heterocyclic Amines during Frying. *J.Agric.Food Chem.*, Vol. 52, pp. 7561-7566.

Pfau, W. & Skog, K. (2004). Exposure to β-carbolines norharman and harman. *J Chromatogr. B*, Vol. 802, pp. 115-126.

Report on Carcinogens. National Toxicology Program. (2011). 12th ed. US Department of Health and Human Services, Public Health Services, Washington DC.

Rich, K.J.; Murray, B.P.; Lewis, I.; Rendell, N.B.; Davies, D.S.; Gooderham, N.J.; & Boobis, A.R. N-Hydroxy-MeIQx is the major microsomal oxidation product of the dietary carcinogen MeIQx with human liver. (1992). *Carcinogenesis*, Vol. 13, pp. 2221-2226.

Ristic, A.; Cichna, M. & Sontag, G. Determination of less polar heterocyclic aromatic amines in standardised beef extracts and cooked meat consumed in Austria by liquid chromatography and fluorescence detection. (2004). *J.Chromatogr.B*, Vol. *802,* pp. 87-94.

Rohrmann, S.; Linseisen, J.; Becker, N.; Norat, T.; Sinha, R.; Skeie, G.; Lund, E.; Martinez, C.; Barricarte, A.; Mattisson, I.; Berglund, G.; Welch, A.; Davey, G.; Overvad, K.; Tjonneland, A.; Clavel-Chapelon, F.; Kesse, E.; Lotze, G.; Klipstein-Grobusch, K.; Vasilopoulou, E.; Polychronopoulos, E.; Pala, V.; Celentano, E., Bueno-de-Mesquita, H.B.; Peeters, P.H.M.; Riboli, E. & Slimani, N. (2002). Cooking of meat and fish in Europe--results from the European Prospective Investigation into Cancer and Nutrition (EPIC). *Eur J Clin Nutr*, Vol. 56, pp. 1216-1230.

Salmon, C.P.; Knize, M.G.; Panteleakos, F.N.; Wu, R.W.; Nelson, D.O. & Felton, J.S. (2000). Minimization of heterocyclic amines and thermal inactivation of Escherichia coli in fried ground beef. *J Natl Cancer Inst*, Vol. *92,* pp. 1773-1778.

Salmon, C.P.; Knize, M.G.; Felton, J.S.; Zhao, B. & Seow, A. (2006). Heterocyclic aromatic amines in domestically prepared chicken and fish from Singapore Chinese households. *Food Chem.* Toxicol., Vol. 44, pp. 484-492.

Shah, F. U.; Barri, T.; Jönsson, J. Å. & Skog, K. (2008). Determination of heterocyclic aromatic amines in human urine by hollow-fibre supported liquid membrane extraction and liquid chromatography-ultraviolet detection system. *J. Chromatogr. B.*, Vol. 870, pp. 203-208.

Shin, H.S.; Rodgers, W.J.; Gomaa, E.A.; Strasburg, G.M. & Gray, J.I. (20029. Inhibition of heterocyclic aromatic amine formation in fried ground beef patties by garlic and selected garlic-related sulfur compounds. *J.Food Protect.*, Vol. 65, pp. 1766-1770.

Sinha, R.; Knize, M.G.; Salmon, C.P.; Brown, E.D.; Rhodes, D.; Felton, J.S.; Levander, O.A. and Rothman, N. (1998a). Heterocyclic amine content of pork products cooked by different methods and to varying degrees of doneness. *Food Chem.Toxicol.*, Vol. 36, pp. 289-297.

Sinha, R.; Rothman, N.; Salmon, C.P.; Knize, M.G.; Brown, E.D.; Swanson, C.A.; Rhodes, D.; Rossi, S.; Felton, J.S. & Levander, O.A. (1998b). Heterocyclic amine content in beef cooked by different methods to varying degrees of doneness and gravy made from meat drippings. *Food Chem.Toxicol.*, Vol. 36, pp. 279-287.

Sinha, R.; Kulldorff, M.; Chow, W.H.; Denobile, J. & Rothman, N. (2001) Dietary-Intake of Heterocyclic Amines, Meat-Derived Mutagenic Activity, and Risk of Colorectal Adenomas. *Cancer Epidem.Biomarker.Prev.* Vol. 10, 559-562.

Skog, K.; Steineck, G.; Augustsson, K. & Jägerstad, M. (1995). Effect of Cooking Temperature on the Formation of Heterocyclic Amines in Fried Meat-Products and Pan Residues. *Carcinogenesis* Vol. 16, pp. 861-867.

Skog, K.; Augustsson, K.; Steineck, G.; Stenberg, M.; & Jägerstad, M. (1997). Polar and Nonpolar Heterocyclic Amines in Cooked Fish and Meat- Products and Their Corresponding Pan Residues. *Food Chem.Toxicol.*, Vol. 35, pp. 555-565.

Skog, K.; Johansson, M.A.E.; & Jägerstad, M.I. (1998). Carcinogenic Heterocyclic Amines in Model Systems and Cooked Foods - A Review on Formation, Occurrence and Intake. *Food Chem.Toxicol.*, Vol. 36, pp. 879-896.

Skog, K.; Eneroth, A.; and Svanberg, M. (2003). Effects of different cooking methods on the formation of food mutagens in meat. *Int.J.Food Sci.Technol.*, Vol. 38, pp. 313-323.

Skog, K. & Jägerstad, M. (2006). Minimising the formation of hazardous compounds in foods during heat treatment, In: *Acrylamide and Other Hazardous Compounds in Heat-Treated Foods* ,Skog, K., Alexander J. (Eds.), pp. 407-424,Woodhead Publishing Limited and CRC Press LLC, ISBN 1-84569-01107,Cambridge and Boca Raton.

Sonestedt, E., Ericson, U., Gullberg, B., Skog, K., Olsson, H., & Wirfält, E. (2008). Do both heterocyclic amines and omega-6 polyunsaturated fatty acids contribute to the incidence of breast cancer in postmenopausal women of the Malmoe diet and cancer cohort? *Int.J.Cancer*, Vol. *123*, pp. 1637-1643.

Sugimura, T. (2002). Food and cancer. Toxicology, Vol. 181-182, pp. 17-21.

Sullivan, R.; Peppercorn, J.; Sikora, K.; Zalcberg, J.; Meropol, N. J.; Amir, E.; Khayat, D.; Boyle, P.; Autier, P.; Tannock, I.F, Fojo, T.; Siderov J., Williamson, S.; Camporesi, S.; Gordon McVie J.; Purushotham, A. D.; Naredi, P.; Eggermont, A.; Brennan, M.F.; Steinberg, M. L.; De Ridder, M.; McCloskey, S. A.; Verellen, D.; Roberts, T.; Storme, G.; Hicks R. J; J Ell P.; Hirsch, B. R.; Carbone, D. P.; Schulman, K. A.; Catchpole, P.; Taylor, D.; Geissler, J.; Brinker, N. G., Meltzer, Da.; Kerr, D.; & Aapro, M. (2011). Delivering affordable cancer care in high-income countries *Lancet Oncol.*, Vol. *12*, pp. 933-980.

Tai, C.Y.; Lee, K.H. & Chen, B.H. (2001). Effects of various additives on the formation of heterocyclic amines in fried fish fibre. *Food Chem.*, Vol. *75*, pp. 309-316.

Tareke E.; Rydberg P.; Karlsson, P.; Eriksson, S & Tornqvist, M. (2002). Analysis of acrylamide, a carcinogen formed in heated foodstuffs. *J Agric Food Chem*; Vol. 50, pp. 4998–5006.

Tehrani, K.A.; Kersiene, M.; Adams, A.; Venskutonis, R. & De Kimpe, N. (2002).Thermal degradation studies of glucose/glycine melanoidins. *J. Agric. Food Chem.*, Vol. 50, pp. 4062-4068.

Teixidó E.; Santos F.J.; Puignou, L.& Galceran M.T. (2006). Analysis of 5-hydroxymethylfurfural in foods by gas chromatography–mass spectrometry. *J. Chromatogr A*, , Vol. 1135, pp. 85-90.

Toribio, F.; Puignou, L.; & Galceran, M.T. (1999). Evaluation of different cleanup procedures for the analysis of heterocyclic aromatic-amines in a lyophilized meat extract. *J.Chromatogr.A*, Vol. 836, 223-233.

Toribio, F.; Busquets, R.; Puignou, L. & Galceran, M.T. (2007).Heterocyclic amines in griddled beef steak analysed using a single extract clean-up procedure. *Food Chem.Toxicol.*, Vol. 45, pp. 667-675.

Tran, N.L., Salmon, C.P., Knize, M.G., & Colvin, M.E. (2002). Experimental and simulation studies of heat flow and heterocyclic amine mutagen/carcinogen formation in pan-fried meat patties. *Food Chem.Toxicol.*, Vol. 40, pp. 673-684.

Tricker, A.R.; Kumar, R.; Siddiqi, M.; Khuroo, M.S.; & Preussmann, R. (1991). Endogenous formation of N-nitrosamines from piperazine and their urinary excretion following anthelmintic treatment with piperazine citrate. *Carcinogenesis*, Vol. *12*, pp. 1595-1599.

Tsen, S.Y.; Ameri, F.; & Smith, J.S. (2006).Effects of rosemary extracts on the reduction of heterocyclic amines in beef patties. *J.Food Sci.*, Vol. *71*, C469-C473.

Turesky, R.J.; Rossi, S.C.; Welti, D.H.; Lay, J.O.; Jr. & Kadlubar, F.F.(1992). Characterization of DNA adducts formed in vitro by reaction of N-hydroxy-2-amino-3-methylimidazo[4,5-f]quinoline and N-hydroxy-2-amino-3,8-dimethylimidazo[4,5-f]quinoxaline at the C-8 and N2 atoms of guanine. *Chem Res Toxicol*, *5*, pp. 479-490.

Turesky, R.J. & Vouros, P. (2004). Formation and analysis of heterocyclic aromatic amine-DNA adducts in vitro and in vivo. *J.Chromatogr.B*, Vol. 802, pp. 155-166.

Turesky, R.J. (2006). Mechanisms of carcinogenicity of heterocyclic amines In: Skog, K., Alexander J. (Eds.), pp. 247-274,Woodhead Publishing Limited and CRC Press LLC, ISBN 1-84569-01107,Cambridge and Boca Raton .

Turesky, R.J.; Goodenough, A.K.; Ni, W.; McNaughton, L.; LeMaster, D.M.; Holland, R.D.; Wu, R.W. & Felton, J.S. (2007). Identification of 2-amino-1,7-dimethylimidazo[4,5-*g*]quinoxaline: an abundant mutagenic heterocyclic aromatic amine formed in cooked beef. *Chem. Res. Toxicol.*, Vol. *20*, pp. 520-530.

Warzecha, L.; Janoszka, B.; Blaszczyk, U.; Strozyk, M.; Bodzek, D. & Dobosz, C. (2004). Determination of heterocyclic aromatic amines (HAs) content in samples of household-prepared meat dishes. *J.Chromatogr.B*, Vol. 802, pp. 95-106.

Widmark, E.M.P. (1939). Presence of cancer-producing substances in roasted food. *Nature*, Vol. 143, pp. 984.

Wong, K.Y.; Su, J.; Knize, M.G.; Koh, W.P. & Seow, A. (2005).Dietary exposure to heterocyclic amines in a Chinese population. *Nutr. Cancer*, Vol. 52, pp. 147-155.

World Health Organization. (2004). The 10 leading causes of death by broad income group. Fact sheet. N° 310, November 2008.

Zhao, K.; Murray, S.; Davies, D.S.; Boobis, A.R. & Gooderham, N.J. (1994). Metabolism of the food-derived mutagen and carcinogen 2-amino-1- methyl-6-phenylimidazo[4,5-*b*]pyridine (PhIP) by human liver- microsomes. *Carcinogenesis*, Vol. 15, pp. 1285-1288.

Zimmerli, B.; Rhyn, P.; Zöller, O.; & Schlatter, J. (2001). Occurrence of Heterocyclic Aromatic-Amines in the Swiss Diet - Analytical Method, Exposure Estimation and Risk Assessment. *Food Addit.Contam.*, Vol. 18, pp. 533-551.

Zöchling, S. & Murkovic, M. (2002).Formation of the heterocyclic amine PhIP: identification of precursors and intermediates. *Food Chem.*, Vol. 79, pp125-134.